OSTEOPOROSIS

THE LONG ROAD BACK

OSTEOPOROSIS

THE LONG ROAD BACK

•

One woman's story

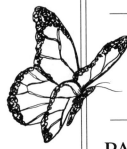

—— • ——

PAMELA HORNER

University of Ottawa Press
Ottawa • London • Paris

Canadian Cataloguing in Publication Data

Horner, Pamela, 1927–
Osteoporosis: the long road back

Includes index.
Bibliography: p.
ISBN 0-7766-0226-8

1. Horner, Pamela, 1927– . 2. Osteoporosis —
Patients — Biography. 3. Osteoporosis — Patients —
Rehabilitation. 4. Osteoporosis — Prevention.
I. Title.

RC931.O73H67 1989   616.7'1   C89-090086-8

© University of Ottawa Press, 1989
Printed and bound in Canada
ISBN 0-7766-0226-8

UNIVERSITÉ 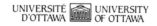 UNIVERSITY
D'OTTAWA   OF OTTAWA

Text and cover design: Peggy Heath
Cover photograph: Heidi Thompson

It is imperative that readers obtain approval from their personal physicians
before adopting procedures outlined in this book. The author, publisher, and
doctors quoted take no responsibility for improper use or misinterpretation
of material contained herein.

Dedicated to the memory of
Lindy Fraser
founder of the first self-help group for osteoporosis

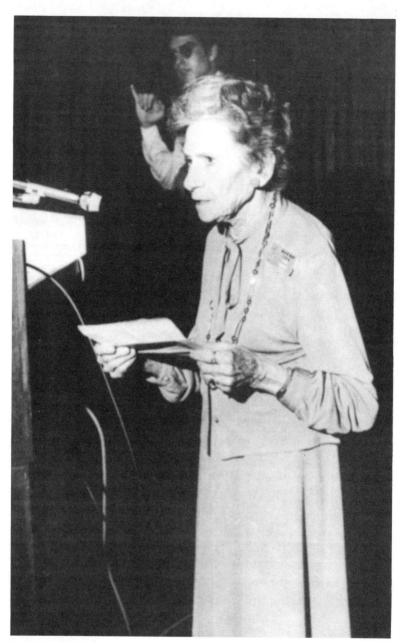

Lindy Fraser

Contents

Figures and Tables

Preface

Early in 1982, at age 54, I became almost totally incapacitated from osteoporotic spinal damage. I was determined to find out all I could about this condition which I had never heard of until it struck me down. My husband, Bill, scoured the library for material. While he found numerous treatises on back ailments in general, there was little information on osteoporosis. Those books that did devote the odd paragraph to the subject concluded that it was part of the aging process and that little could be done in the way of prevention or treatment. This wasn't good enough for me. I questioned my doctors at length. I wrote to the Osteoporosis Society of Canada, and tracked down leads from items on radio and television. Eventually I accumulated a large file on osteoporosis which, together with my own experience, constitutes the backbone of this book.

At the same time as I was compiling my material, the popular press began to focus more on this insidious disorder so that now osteoporosis is well on its way to becoming a household word. Why then is a book such as this still important? There are several reasons. While articles on the subject have proliferated, they cannot go into great detail. There is a need for a more in-depth work, for a comprehensive summary of causes, effects, preventive measures and recent medical advances and, perhaps most important, for advice on dealing with the ravages of the disease from someone who has had personal experience.

Some people may think it presumptuous of a layperson to write in such detail on a medical topic. To allay their misgivings I have thoroughly documented the medical references and personally contacted the doctors who are quoted extensively in Chapters 2 and 3. A qualified dietician has verified the medical accuracy of Chapter 5. Where opinions or advice arise from my personal experience, I have stated so.

My purpose was to put together a book that would be helpful to the layperson, but would not be entirely subjective. In defining osteoporosis, its causes and effects, and current research and treatment, I have tried as much as possible to avoid "doctor talk" and to put such anatomical explanations as are necessary in terms the layperson can understand. This was at times difficult, as much of my research material was couched in medical phraseology. If here and there, primarily in quotations, technical terms have crept in, I hope the reader will bear with me.

At the outset I did not visualize such an extensive work. My original intention was to write a short article on my own experience with osteoporosis. But when I began to seek information from medical professionals, the floodgates opened, and so much material poured in that my article began to take on book-like proportions. Had I realized at the outset that the project would send me winging across the country to interviews and symposia and involve months of sifting through medical data, I might have lost heart. I received so much encouragement from so many quarters, however, that I felt obliged to persevere.

I must express my heartfelt thanks to those many individuals without whose help this project would never have reached fruition.

Foremost among these is Lindy Fraser of Ottawa, founder of the first self-help group for osteoporosis in the world. I was saddened to hear of her death in January 1989. More in Chapter 7 about this amazing lady, to whose memory the book is dedicated. Suffice it to say here that without her encouragement and the avenues she opened, the book would never have been written.

It was through one of Lindy's "babies," the Regina Osteoporosis Group, that I learned of Barry Ashpole and Associates of Toronto. Barry Ashpole, in his then capacity as Public Relations consultant for Sandoz Canada Inc., had for some years been concerned with raising the level of public awareness of osteoporosis. For some two years he kept a steady stream of factual data flowing into my mailbox. And his encouraging phone calls more than once served to "whet my almost blunted purpose."

Pauline Witherly-Manuel, President of Ostop Ottawa, was very helpful in supplying current addresses and providing liaison with Lindy Fraser.

The British Columbia Dairy Foundation supplied much of the research material for Chapter 5. Thanks to Patricia Lippert, Nutrition Educator with that organization, for her co-operation.

Many of the doctors quoted took the time to write encouraging letters which were indeed heartening. To them my deepest appreciation.

I'm grateful also to my artist son, Jim, who took time out during his Christmas vacation to sketch the diagrams while I performed my exercise routine.

And last, but certainly not least, special thanks to my husband, Bill, whose faith and constant encouragement kept me going. He was also a great help in researching, compiling tables, and photo-copying data, to say nothing of persevering without complaint in the face of dustballs under the bed, leftovers for dinner, and living with a frequently harried wife!

Introduction

If you are a post-menopausal woman, the chances are one in four that you harbour within your body a bone robber, called osteoporosis, which for years has been undermining the foundations of your skeletal system. Osteoporosis is a major medical problem that affects millions of people, particularly women over the age of 50. It is estimated that more than 800,000 Canadian women have been diagnosed as osteoporotic, and that some 20 million women in the United States who are 50 or over are likely to have radiographically detectable evidence of osteopenia (decreased bone mass). The annual medical costs incurred in the United States for treatment of osteoporosis and related fractures exceed $6 billion.

The bone robber may remain undetected in your body until, by slowly depleting the mineral content, it has reduced your bone mass by as much as 30 per cent. And you, the victim, left with the brittle bones of the osteoporotic, will be subject to fractures of wrist or hip at the slightest trauma. You may also suffer wedge or crush fractures of one or several vertebrae (often five will collapse to a point where they occupy the space formerly taken by three). This causes the unsightly "dowager's hump" and an attendant height loss and realignment of bodily structures which can have devastating results. The accompanying pain, usually associated with the back area, can be completely incapacitating.

Now, suppose a robber were repeatedly breaking into your home and stealing your valuables. You would at once take countermeasures. You'd make sure you kept your doors locked, perhaps even install a burglar alarm. But if that same robber went undetected, if you didn't miss the valuables being stolen, you would have no cause for increased vigilance. This is the dilemma that confronts potential victims of the bone robber—the need to take precautionary measures long before the damage becomes apparent.

It was with the dual purpose of convincing women, particularly young women, that they should look to their defences, and of helping those already suffering the ravages of attack, that I embarked on this project. I have tried to write in an optimistic vein, stressing the positive, so that other sufferers in search of information may not meet with the discouraging blank wall I initially encountered.

I sincerely hope that my readers, be they known or potential victims of the bone robber, will take the message to heart. I do not claim you can banish the culprit, but I am convinced that by following the relatively simple preventive and curative measures outlined here, you can do much to hogtie him. If even a few readers are helped to this end—if the potential victim looks to her defences, if the acute sufferer finds cause to hope and courage to persevere—then I will have achieved my goal.

Chapter 1
Metamorphosis:
A Personal Story

July 1983. Bill and I stand hand in hand at Inspiration Point above the Grand Canyon in Yellowstone National Park. We have spent two glorious weeks camping in the park, tracking its awesome wonders, hiking its quiet trails. That trip marked the high point of my return to relative normalcy from the abyss of despair and incapacity that had characterized my life during the greater part of the two preceding years.

But let's begin at the beginning—admittedly not an easy task when dealing with osteoporosis, since the beginning is all but impossible to pin down. In my case, it may have been at the moment of conception when a certain gene marker predisposed me genetically to the condition. This is speculation, but not implausible, and will be discussed further in Chapter 2. The first manifestations which led my doctor to a vague suspicion that I might be osteoporotic came in July 1981.

EARLY WARNING

One day that summer, in an effort to contract my diaphragm and dislodge a piece of steak lodged in my throat, it appeared that Bill had squeezed too hard and broken a rib (mine, not his!). This almost spontaneous fracture, coupled with the fact that I'd fractured a toe a year or so before, made the doctor just suspicious enough to question my calcium intake. On being assured, however, that I was a milk drinker, ate a balanced diet, and did regular calisthenics and a lot of walking, he dismissed the idea of osteoporosis, and I went my merry way.

In September of that year I fell and broke my wrist. Ensuing X-rays exhibited some fuzziness indicating possible loss of bone density. In mid-November, after the cast came off, the general practitioner referred me to an internist for possible diagnosis of osteoporosis. This specialist seemed skeptical at first. He questioned me closely as to whether I felt the various broken bones were justified by the force of the accidents that caused them. He was extremely interested and concerned, however, to learn that for 18 years I had been on a thyroid hormone supplement (Thyroxin 0.4 mg a day). I gathered from him (and have subsequently confirmed from numerous sources) that an excess of thyroid hormone can have a deleterious effect on bone.

A month went by after this examination with no word from either doctor. When I called to enquire, I was sent for a T.4 (thyroid hormone) blood test. It showed, as had others on previous occasions, that I was within the normal range, but at the high end of that range. The medication was cut to 0.3 mg a day. No more was said about osteoporosis, so I assumed that there was no evidence of this condition.

In early January 1982, however, I began to have serious back problems. I'd had the odd session of back pain before, maybe two or three times in the previous couple of years, but it had always cleared up on its own. I wasn't unduly alarmed, therefore, when I felt a twinge as I bent over the deep freeze juggling boxes and bags from one side to the other. That was on a Friday. By the following Monday, I was in such agony that I decided to seek medical help.

I went to the phone, still undecided whether to call my G.P. or a chiropractor. I decided on the latter, which proved to have been a bad mistake. I don't mean to denigrate chiropractors in general. They may help a lot of people, including back pain sufferers. In fact, personal testimony to this effect from several friends led to my decision to seek chiropractic aid. But some two months later when I found out what was wrong with my back, I realized that it certainly couldn't be helped by spinal manipulation—quite the reverse, in fact. The last thing my poor calcium-depleted vertebrae needed was someone trying to pound them into shape.

Still, in my ignorance, I paid several visits to the chiropractor, and there did seem to be some slight improvement. But one

4

morning in mid-February (some six weeks after the initial attack) I awoke barely able to struggle out of bed. I decided to give up on the chiropractor and made an appointment with my G.P.

The doctor referred me to a physiotherapist, explaining that most back pain is muscular in origin and responds to rest and therapy. I am sure that is true but, in my case, this treatment did no good at all. The mere mechanics of getting to and from the therapist's office and of climbing onto the table caused excruciating pain. And the practitioner, obviously underestimating the degree of disability, would blithely instruct me to "turn on your left side, now the right side," demanding the near impossible of me. After two such traumatic visits, I phoned my doctor's office requesting an X-ray. I felt it was high time they found out just what they were treating me for. Another two weeks passed before I got the X-rays.

Meanwhile I continued to suffer acutely. Getting in and out of bed was so agonizing that I spent most nights sitting in a chair with a heating pad at my back. I still dragged myself to work at my part-time receptionist job, although how I did so is a mystery, even to me.

In early March, however, when the X-ray results arrived, they spelled the end of my working days for a long time to come. They showed an alarming decrease in bone mass and several compacted vertebrae. The internist, obviously extremely concerned, put me directly into hospital for a series of tests. It was imperative to seek the cause of the extreme calcium depletion, unusual for my relatively young age (I was then 54). Some of the possible implications (I'll not go into them here) were terrifying.

HOSPITALIZATION AND DIAGNOSIS

I spent 12 days in hospital, during which time I established a routine of sorts that I could live with, although I was only truly comfortable flat on my back with several pillows under my knees. And there was the eternal problem of getting in and out of bed. I usually stayed up during the morning, walking as much as I could. I wore out the pockets of two housecoats by pressing my hands in them and pulling the garment tightly over my sore back (my substitute for the support girdle that had been mentioned, but not yet prescribed). After lunch I'd lie down until visiting hours were over, then get up and walk or sit until after supper.

I slept badly, mostly due to the difficulty of turning over, although the raised sides on the bed helped somewhat. By grasping the bars, I could make my arms take much of the strain of turning.

Such was the almost unvarying routine of my 12-day sojourn in hospital. Of course there were such added discomforts as near daily extraction of blood for testing, a 24-hour urine collection, and additional X-rays. During my stay in hospital, my thyroid supplement was reduced to 0.1 mg a day, and, in the last few days, the regimen of calcium, fluoride, estrogen, and vitamin D therapy began. It was determined that I suffered from "idiopathic osteoporosis" (osteoporosis not resulting from any other condition). Tests for all the more devastating possibilities had proved negative.

On the tenth day, an orthopedic specialist appeared, asked a few questions, ran his hand over my spine, had me raise my legs to rule out any nerve involvement, and prescribed the long-awaited lumbo-sacral support. I had suffered much trepidation about this garment, as a nurse had already shown me one that resembled a medieval torture implement. When a therapist brought the girdle for fitting, however, I was relieved to see that it was not unlike the ones Mom used to wear, except for two contoured steel slats running down either side of the spine. To one used to freedom from all such devices it was an inconvenience, but it did, and still does, provide welcome support for my back.

The therapist also prescribed a few mild exercises such as the pelvic tilt and leg bending, and showed me how to get in and out of bed with the least amount of strain. This was the only advice relating to back pain that I received during my hospital sojourn.

In retrospect I realize that my doctors were primarily concerned with arresting the alarming calcium drain, seeking its cause, and treating it, rather than merely alleviating the symptoms. In so doing, they moved with a speed and efficiency for which I am grateful. Nevertheless, it was disconcerting to arrive home after 12 days in hospital with the same incapacitating back pain and the same seemingly insurmountable problem of how to cope.

COPING ON THE HOME FRONT

My first step was to select a rocking chair from the array that Bill had brought home on approval. I chose a platform rocker with an almost straight back, a minimum of padding, and wide arm rests. When ensconced in it with a heating pad at my back and a stool for my feet, I was almost pain free.

But I couldn't spend all my time in the old rocking chair. There was still the problem of where to sleep. The first couple of nights I opted for the living room sofa because I could curl my spine against the back of the couch for support. When the home therapist called, however, she outlawed the couch because it was too soft.

This sunny-dispositioned Irish woman was the most helpful person the medical profession had yet offered in terms of dealing with the pain. She showed me how to "log-roll" from side to side to avoid the painful twisting motion, and how to use my arms for support in getting in and out of bed. She surveyed the house with a critical eye, poked and prodded the beds, and approved of the firmness of our queen-sized mattress. She brought a commode with arms to fit over the toilet, and another to stand beside the bed for night use. She prescribed a few more mild exercises and forbade me to sit for more than 15 minutes at a time.

This last advice put me in a quandary. The doctors were insistent that I keep on the move as much as possible because calcium loss accelerates when you're lying down. The therapists all agree, however, that the only way to cure back pain with acute muscle spasm is to stay in bed, preferably on your back with a bolster under the knees. Faced with this dilemma, I had to work out a compromise.

While pain and general weakness forced me to bed for the greater part of the day, I interspersed these rests with "walk-abouts" through living room, dining room, kitchen and hall. When sitting to watch television I'd do one of these route marches whenever an ad came on, which conformed fairly well to the admonition not to sit for more than 15 minutes at a time. Public Broadcasting did present some difficulty in this regard, there being no commercials!

Every afternoon I'd struggle into the loose, A-line dress which became my uniform during this period, in preparation for a short walk outside when Bill returned from work. At first I was able to make it only two or three houses down the street, but I extended the distance by a few yards each day. It was over a month before I could get all the way around the block.

We must have presented quite a spectacle—with my one hand clasped tightly in Bill's, the other wielding my trusty cane, and my back bent over at a near 45-degree angle. I'm sure I must have looked like Bill's mother, if not his grandmother. I know that's how I felt. These walks were extremely painful both physically and psychologically. Even my legs hurt, which I supposed was due partly to the long period of relative inactivity, but which I later concluded had a lot to do with the drastic realignment of my spinal structure.

Evenings were spent alternately lying in bed and sitting up to watch television or visit with friends and family. I usually retired for the night at about 10:00 p.m. I slept reasonably well despite waking a few times during the night to execute the convoluted procedure involved in turning from one side to the other.

This almost unvarying routine continued for some four months. Of course there were occasional diversions when friends dropped in offering moral support, along with casserole dishes and other goodies to help Bill in the battle of the home front. These were necessary because I was unable to do any housework or cooking during this period. Lifting even a litre carton of milk was out of the question. It was all I could do to brush my teeth and hair because raising my arms even to shoulder height was extremely painful.

During the second month of this routine, there was the added variation of twice-weekly visits to the hospital physiotherapy department. Luckily our 18-year-old son Gordon, a college student, was able to work the chauffeuring duties into his busy schedule. The fact that he was still living at home, and that we had a two-week visit from our daughter in April, helped relieve the pressure on Bill and keep us both sane.

PSYCHOLOGICAL ASPECTS

The psychological trauma associated with the acute phase of osteoporosis is an aspect seldom touched on in the literature. But in my case it was a major problem. It was a bitter pill to be so utterly dependent on my family for the basic needs of life. For example, I couldn't shower without assistance, and Bill had to wash my hair at the kitchen sink where, by leaning on the counter, I could just manage to get my head under the tap.

This almost total helplessness made me terrified of being alone for any length of time. One day when I was lying in bed, a sudden storm blew up. I couldn't close the windows or rescue items I heard being smashed on the patio. I just had to lie there and pray that the damage wouldn't be serious. And when I first ventured outside on my own, I had an almost pathological fear of falling.

Then there was the dramatic height loss and resultant rearranging of my figure to deal with. When the spine shrinks so drastically, it causes the abdomen to protrude in a most unsightly fashion and the waistline completely disappears. This, coupled with a noticeable curvature of the upper spine, made me dread looking in the mirror. It was disconcerting, to say the least, to see the face and figure of my aged mother reflected there in place of the slim, straight me of a few short months ago. Even now, when exercise and increasing strength have enabled me to straighten up considerably, I shudder when I catch sight of my walking profile reflected in a store window. I can only liken it to that of a chicken which leads with its head!

Finding clothes to conform to this structural realignment was another problem. Any close-fitting garment was now three or four inches (7 to 10 cm) too small around the middle, and everything that was still wearable had to be shortened. It was a constant trial to have to remodel or buy clothes that would present a reasonably neat appearance.

Another psychological aspect which was perhaps the most difficult to deal with was my uncertainty about the future. The doctors were understandably vague because it would be some months before they'd be able to determine whether the calcium drain had been arrested. And there would probably be no perceptible increase in bone mass for at least a year, if ever. In my darkest moments I'd visualize all my bones disintegrating until I dissolved into an amorphous mass and slithered out under the door!

Mornings were the worst. I'd awake between 5:00 and 6:00 a.m. with a leaden feeling in the pit of my stomach. Not wishing to wake Bill who was sleeping in the next room (another "downer" after 30 years of sharing our double bed), I'd lie quietly for an hour or so, wondering if the nightmare would ever end. When breakfast was ready, I'd creep out to my rocker and force as much food as I could past the lump in my throat. Eating at any time was no great pleasure during this period, but in the morning it took an effort of will.

9

Not that I was in a constant state of depression. In more rational moments I was able to adopt a fairly positive attitude, particularly as slowly—oh so very slowly—I became a bit more mobile.

My saving graces during this period were my insatiable appetite for books and the constant companionship of CBC (Canadian Broadcasting Corporation) radio. If I could remember all the bits of miscellany that diverted me during those months, I'd be a world champion at Trivial Pursuit! At first I confined my reading mostly to novels which were light, both literally and figuratively. But as I got stronger and became more curious about my condition, I began to devour all the literature I could find on back conditions in general, and osteoporosis in particular.

The main message of several books by orthopedic specialists was the need for back patients to perform certain exercises regularly. I took this advice to heart, and over the next year I gradually developed a more rigorous exercise program to which I credit, in large measure, my present near-normal mobility. More about exercise and the extreme caution with which osteoporotics must proceed in Chapter 6. Suffice it to say here that performing this daily exercise routine produced positive effects both physically and psychologically. The exercise program, coupled with gradually increased walking distances, and the constant support of family and friends, combined to pull me through the psychological trauma. Most doctors today recognize that the well-being of the mind is essential to recovering from a physical disability.

SUMMARY OF ACUTE PHASE

The following is a month by month summary of the year which I call my acute phase of osteoporotic disability.

January 1982
Intermittent acute back pain. Turn to chiropractor for help. No perceptible improvement.

February 1982
A completely disabling attack. Seek medical advice. Still working 20 hours a week at office job, but suffering acutely.

March 1982
X-rays reveal acute osteopenia (decreased bone mass). Hospital-

ized for tests. Idiopathic osteoporosis diagnosed. No alleviation of back pain. Calcium, fluoride, estrogen, and vitamin D prescribed.

April 1982
Continue routine at home. Walking distances gradually increased.

May 1982
Started in-hospital therapy sessions twice weekly. Improvement very slow. Still almost completely incapacitated.

June 1982
Repeat of blood and urine tests show calcium drain apparently arrested. Battery of X-rays reveal no improvement in bone mass, but no further deterioration. Internist pleased with my general condition and increasing mobility. Medication unchanged and support girdle still a must.

July 1982
My spirits improve because my husband Bill, a teacher, will be home for two months. Since it is now not so vital that his sleep be undisturbed, we resume sharing our double bed, another "upper." Starting to do light housework. Walking distance increased to about half a mile (800 m). Try swimming, but painful to straighten legs in prone position even in water.

August 1982
Late in the month, decide I am well enough to try a short trip to Victoria. Only a van, outfitted for camping, with firm mattress enables me to tackle this project, as I can rest en route. Find swimming a bit easier in heated pool after a session in the Jacuzzi. Still don't have to fake to let four-year-old granddaughter win race across pool! Trip a positive factor, even if physically quite tiring.

September 1982
Am able to cope with the "downers" of Bill's return to work and Gordon leaving the nest to attend University of Victoria. By now am doing most of the housework and am entirely comfortable lying or sitting as long as I maintain the proper posture for back patients (see Chapter 4). Walking still not entirely natural or comfortable.

October 1982
Am able to help with canning, drying, and freezing produce for winter as long as someone else does any lifting involved. Can even do a bit of gardening sitting on a low hassock.

November 1982
Begin early to get ready for Christmas, as I can stand up to only abbreviated shopping excursions. Beginning to feel time hanging heavy and decide I'm well enough to go back to work at least on a trial basis.

December 1982
Boost to morale of working outside the home. Welcome from staff and clients more than compensates for sore back at the end of each shift. Christmas is a mixed blessing. All the family is home (we are nine in all). Great to have everyone here, but tiring. Manage to adhere to exercise and rest regimen throughout the holiday.

January 1983
Mixed feelings when the mass exodus takes place. Miss them all, but know it is good for me to resume "the even tenor of my ways" after a hectic two weeks.

February 1983
Complete X-rays of spine and long bones show no perceptible improvement in bone density. The relative ease with which I am able to perform the gyrations involved in this procedure, however, assures me that I am vastly improved.

Progress from now on is steady, but less dramatic.

By the summer of 1984, some two and a half years after the onset of osteoporotic symptoms, I was able to walk five miles or more with a couple of short rests along the way. I had resumed all household tasks including vacuuming and such outdoor jobs as lawn mowing and gardening, the latter mostly from a kneeling or squatting position. Heavy work such as digging was, and still is, out of the question. I still have to pace myself and rest for an hour or so during the day. My back continues to be weak and sore at times, but there is none of the excruciating pain and immobility of the acute phase.

I know I'll always have to be careful and observe the rules for back patients as outlined in Chapter 4. The exercise program (now reduced to one half-hour session a day) will always be necessary. It has become as much a part of my morning routine as brushing my teeth.

I have completely come to terms with the degree of disability that I must live with. I know I'll never recover the lost height. I'll never run or jump again. I'll always feel acutely the slightest lump in a mattress (Bill likens me to the fabled princess who could feel a pea through several mattresses!). I'll never recover my girlish figure, and I've managed to adjust my wardrobe accordingly. In short, I can now "accentuate the positive" and be thankful for the things I can do, rather than constantly lament the things I can't.

And there are even some positive aspects to the whole traumatic experience. I've gained a greater empathy with the elderly and handicapped. My outlook on life has become more philosophical. And, best of all, I've come to know a deeper love and respect for my husband of 30 years.

Without Bill's unfailing support I know I wouldn't have recovered to the extent I have. He never complained at having the entire load of running house and garden thrust upon him. He was never too tired to take my hand for our daily walk. He drove me to and from doctor, therapist, and medical laboratory. He even helped me shop for dresses. In short, throughout the whole ordeal he proved to be a rare gem.

How appropriate, then, that Bill should be by my side that July day in 1983 as I stood on Inspiration Point drinking in the wonder of Yellowstone Canyon and marvelling at the very fact of our being there. Looking back to my total incapacity of the previous year, I felt that I had truly achieved a metamorphosis.

PERSONAL UPDATE

As considerable time has passed since the completion of the first draft of my manuscript, a brief outline of my progress during the intervening years is in order.

There has been no perceptible change in my overall condition since 1984. All medication was discontinued after a period of three years on estrogen and vitamin D therapy and four years on sodium fluoride. I still make sure that I get adequate vitamin D through diet and exposure to sunshine, with a modest supplement (multivitamin or liver-oil capsule) during the winter months. Also, I continue to be acutely conscious of the calcium factor, taking a minimal supplement from time to time when circumstances, such as travelling, do not permit adequate dietary intake.

My general health remains good, though I seem to tire more easily than I would consider normal for a woman of 60. I presume this is to be expected with the added load extensive spinal damage puts on the musculature.

Nevertheless, I was able to accompany Bill on a sabbatical leave in Europe during the 1985-1986 school year, although it was with some trepidation that I set out on this adventure. Armed with a letter from my doctor, which I hoped would preclude our being thrown in jail should some overly zealous customs officer happen upon my travelling medicine kit, we flew off to London in September 1985. There we purchased an aged Volkswagen camper which saw us through many adventures in foreign driving.

I discovered during this holiday that I could stand up to greater exertion than I had previously attempted. Though my back was often crying out by the end of the day, a good rest with a couple of pillows under my knees always put it to rights. I never had to resort to pain medication. Bill, as usual, was patient with my need for adequate rest. And because we were, for the most part, self-catering in homes or apartments, we were free to set our own schedule. The most difficult periods (never more than a week or two at any one stretch) were when we stayed at different small hotels or bed and breakfast establishments each evening. I was invariably over-tired before we got bedded down, and sometimes the mattresses left much to be desired. I soon learned, however, to test them before we took a room and to ask for a board if necessary, which most landlords were quite willing to provide.

I still continued to do my exercises each morning, and sight-seeing involved miles of walking most days which was probably beneficial if sometimes exhausting. On the whole, this eight-month experience was most rewarding, especially considering that only three years earlier I'd been almost completely incapacitated.

Coming home from our ''dream trip'' was a bit of a letdown. A further blow came when I learned that reorganization at my place of employment had phased out my part-time job. This made me realize anew just how strong is the link between mental and physical well-being. I was so devastated, weepy and mopey, that

I began to fear for my general state of health. Eventually I decided to seek fulfilment through volunteer work. This helped a great deal, but my self-image, wounded by enforced retirement, was slow to heal.

After Bill retired (voluntarily!) in July 1987, we both became involved in so many projects that boredom was no longer an issue. Quite the reverse, in fact. Travelling is still a high priority when the budget permits, as is enrolment in courses at the local college, and participation in Elder Hostel programs.

After a down year, I think I can say I'm back on track. And I still feel the best advice I can offer fellow osteoporotics is to keep as busy as your health permits at whatever projects interest you.

Chapter 2
The Nature
of the Beast

In this chapter we will first define osteoporosis and examine who is most likely to fall prey to the disease. Following this are the effects—in particular curvature of the spine—and, finally, the early symptoms of osteoporosis.

WHAT IS OSTEOPOROSIS?

Literally, the term means porous bones, a condition resulting from progressive loss of bone mass over a period of years. It has lately become accepted that there are two types of osteoporosis, both displaying diminished bone mass, but with different patterns of sex and age distribution and fracture location.

> Type I *osteoporosis occurs six times as often in women, usually between the ages of 55 and 75 . . . the fractures usually occur in the spinal vertebrae (the classic crush fracture) or the wrist.* Type II *osteoporosis which has "only" twice as many female as male victims, is a disease of older people, ages 70 to 85 . . . the most common fracture sites are the hips and other long bones.*
> (Smith, Wendy, *Osteoporosis—How to Prevent the Brittle Bone Disease.* Simon & Schuster, N.Y. 1985, p. 23).

Although the causes of the two types of osteoporosis are somewhat similar, and although most of the advice I offer would apply to either, I will be referring mainly to Type I, or "postmenopausal" osteoporosis.

Bones get their strength from a structure of flexible protein fibres combined with hard calcium phosphate crystals. Bone is not a static material. Throughout life it is constantly remodelled by cells which build up and break down. One could liken the process to that of keeping a brick wall in a state of repair. Your skeleton, like the wall, is only in trouble if the number of bricks broken down exceeds the number replaced with new ones.

Up to about age 35 this remodelling process usually results in a net increase in bone mass. But after that age, more bone is removed than is replaced, so that a net loss occurs. This process occurs in both sexes, but because women usually have less bone mass to begin with, and because post-menopausal women lose the protective effect of estrogen, it is this latter category that is most at risk.

Another analogy is suggested by Dr. Frederick S. Kaplan, Chief, Division of Metabolic Bone Diseases, University of Pennsylvania School of Medicine*:

> *The skeleton is not only an adaptable and well-articulated frame, but also a dynamic mineral reserve bank in which the body stores its calcium and phosphorus. . . . The cells of the bone . . . function as both construction workers and metabolic bankers, dual roles that often conflict.*
>
> *When the assets of the skeletal bank fall below normal . . . osteoporosis results. Osteoporosis is a generic term, referring to a skeletal state of decreased mass per unit volume of normally mineralized bone. Osteoporosis is the most common skeletal disorder in the world, and second only to arthritis as a leading cause of musculo-skeletal morbidity in the elderly.*

A word of explanation regarding Dr. Kaplan's reference to metabolic bankers is in order. Calcium, the chief element we are concerned with, is required not only to maintain bone density, but also for various body processes associated with metabolism. If you aren't getting sufficient calcium, or if, for some reason,

*Quotes from Dr. Kaplan are reprinted with permission from *Clinical Symposia* by Frederick S. Kaplan, M.D. Illustrated by Frank H. Netter, M.D. Copyright 1983 CIBA-GEIGY Corporation.

absorption of calcium from the intestine is decreased, the amount needed for these vital metabolic functions will be withdrawn from the bones. The bone robber will be working overtime!

To sum up, then, osteoporosis may be described simply as a decrease in bone mass sufficient to produce "brittle bones," which are subject to fracture with little or no related trauma. It can occur in either sex, but is most prevalent among post-menopausal women.

THOSE MOST AT RISK

Having defined osteoporosis, we will now attempt to determine who is most at risk. Dr. Kaplan writes:

> *The many factors that influence attainment and maintenance of peak bone mass also eventually determine who is at risk of osteoporosis. The person most likely to be affected is a sedentary, postmenopausal white woman with a lifelong dietary calcium deficiency.*

Let's examine these factors individually.

SEDENTARY

This is a vague term, but with reference to bone loss, it could be applied to anyone who isn't following some regular exercise program, be it walking briskly for at least half an hour a day, or following a prescribed regimen of calisthenics. It is important to note that, in order to prevent bone loss, exercises must include those of the weight-bearing variety, e.g., isometrics, walking, running, deep knee bends, racquet sports, etc. According to Dr. Kaplan, "mechanical weight-bearing stress is perhaps the most important exogenous factor affecting bone development and remodelling."

And Dr. Joan Harrison of the Bone and Mineral Metabolism Unit, University of Toronto, states:

> *Perhaps osteoporosis is related to the sedentary occupations or affluent lifestyle of Canadians. With complete inactivity there is profound bone loss. Bone loss occurs with paralysis or with prolonged illness. Even astronauts lose bone during space flight when the forces of gravity are no longer present. . . . It appears that*

19

the strength of our skeletons is maintained by the forces put upon it through physical activity.

Everett L. Smith, Ph.D., Assistant Clinical Professor in the Department of Medicine, University of Wisconsin, reports in *The Physician and Sports Medicine* (March 1982) on various experiments relating physical activity to bone mass. One such study conducted by Donaldson et al. states, in part:

> *A 36-week bed rest study of three young men demonstrated a calcaneus bone mineral content loss of 39%. . . . Rambaut et al. reported similar results in eight subjects immobilized for 24 weeks . . .*

Dr. Smith also quotes studies showing substantial differences in the bone density of the racquet-wielding arm of tennis players and the throwing arm of baseball pitchers compared to that of their other arms.

Another interesting experiment reported by Dr. Smith involved a group of 30 elderly women (18 controls and 12 participants) matched on the basis of age, weight, and degree of ambulation. The control group made no change in their daily activities during the course of the experiment. The other group participated in an exercise program for 30 minutes a day, three days a week for three years. During this 36-month period the control group had a bone mineral content loss of 3.28 per cent, while the group participating in the exercise program exhibited a 2.29 per cent gain.

It is abundantly evident from the foregoing that a sedentary lifestyle greatly increases the risk of osteoporosis.

POST-MENOPAUSAL

Menopause, whether occurring naturally or surgically induced by hysterectomy, often triggers a dramatic decrease in bone mass. It might be well to examine the reasons for this. Dr. Kaplan writes:

> *Sex differences in bone loss are dramatic. At any given age bone mass is greater in men than in women. Moreover, in the decade after age 40 men lose only about .5 to .75% of bone mass yearly, while women lose bone at more than twice that rate . . . following menopause the rate of bone loss in some women may temporarily approach 3% a year.*

Various studies have shown that this alarming loss in bone mass is primarily associated with lack of the female sex hormone, estrogen. Dr. Robert P. Heaney, a professor at the John A. Creighton University, Omaha, Nebraska, reports in this connection:

> *Estrogen affects both the absorption and excretion of calcium . . . for any given intake there is about 14 mg more calcium absorbed daily from the diet in the presence than in the absence of estrogen . . . for any given absorbed intake of calcium, urinary calcium is higher in the absence than in the presence of estrogen. Thus in the absence of estrogen, a woman absorbs calcium less well and excretes it more vigorously. She is losing on both sides of the balance equation.*

WHITE WOMEN

Statistics point to racial and regional differences in the incidence of osteoporosis. In a recently published book, *Osteoporosis: Brittle Bones and the Calcium Crisis* (pp. 36/37), Kathleen Mayes states that the condition is most prevalent in Northern Europe, China and Japan and among the Arctic Inuit of Canada and Alaska, and less common in Africa and Mediterranean countries and among Australian aborigines.

Dr. Joan Harrison lists North America and New Zealand among the regions whose populations are most at risk. She suggests that these regional differences reflect the possible importance of such factors as climate, occupation, environment, genetics, and nutrition.

Other researchers attribute the considerably smaller incidence of osteoporosis among black people to a generally greater bone mass throughout life. But whatever the reason, it is well documented that white women, particularly those of slight build, are a high risk category for osteoporosis. The condition is also more prevalent among women with fair hair and complexion.

CALCIUM DEFICIENCY

Many of my sources point to evidence of an alarming deficiency in calcium intake in the North American adult diet. For example, Dr. B. Lawrence Riggs, Chairman of the Division of Endocrinology and Metabolism, Mayo Medical School, Rochester, Minnesota, states that a normal American diet with no milk products contains about 250 mg of calcium per day, and that most Americans get no more than 500 mg daily. He points to metabolic studies done at Creighton University which show that "premenopausal women lose bone mass when their calcium intake falls below a gram a day. Post-menopausal women lose bone when their intake falls below 1.5 grams, due to less efficient absorption of calcium after menopause."

FACTORS WHICH MAY CONTRIBUTE TO RISK

While it is generally accepted that these factors (sedentary lifestyle, menopause, racial origin, and calcium deficiency) increase the risk of osteoporosis, there are other circumstances which may increase susceptibility. Let's look at these briefly.

DIETARY FACTORS

Excessive Protein Again, I quote Dr. Kaplan:

> *Protein consumption also affects daily calcium requirements as increased protein intake accelerates calcium excretion by the kidney. [In an experimental study] doubling the daily protein intake increased urinary calcium losses by 50%, and the high protein diet common in western industrialized countries may be a major cause of accelerated bone loss in these populations.*

And Dr. Heaney states:

> *Increased protein intake is clearly associated with calcium balance in our patients, as well as in the pioneering work of Linkswiler and Margen and their associates over the years. . . . We saw exactly the same phenomenon as they did—an increase in protein intake is associated with more urinary calcium and negative calcium balance. In other words, protein appears to increase the dietary requirement for calcium.*

Caffeine Dr. Heaney and Dr. Robert Recker, in a 17-year study of 168 women who were between the ages of 36 and 45 at the outset, found that even a moderate amount of caffeine in the diet may be associated with a deterioration in calcium balance, and they add that women who consume a lot of caffeine also seem to consume fewer calcium-rich foods.

Dr. Joan Harrison states that "the excessive intake of caffeine in tea and coffee appears to have an adverse affect on bones."

Dr. P. D. Delmas and Dr. Riggs, of the Mayo Clinic, say "caffeine has a small but real effect on calcium metabolism."

Vitamin D Deficiency Dr. Kaplan:

> *The vitamin D metabolite is the active hormone that helps maintain normal serum calcium and phosphate levels. . . . About half our vitamin D comes from dietary sources and the remainder from an endogenous reaction in the skin stimulated by ultraviolet radiation. Only a few natural foods, such as fish liver oils, contain vitamin D. Most milk sold in the United States (and Canada) is fortified with 400 IU of vitamin D per quart. The elderly are frequently mildly vitamin D deficient. . . . The recommended daily dietary allowance of vitamin D is 400 IU for young adults. For the elderly 800 IU daily is recommended.*

Excess Alcohol and Tobacco Such phrases as "high bone loss is common among heavy drinkers" and "excessive cigarette smoking may be an important factor" appear in the literature. It would seem prudent, therefore, for osteoporotics and those in the high risk category to cut out or, at the very least, curtail consumption of alcohol and tobacco.

GENETIC FACTORS

Dr. Kaplan writes:

> *The cells themselves are endowed with genetic instructions that determine their ability to form, resorb, or maintain bone. These internal genetic factors may be critically important in the ultimate understanding of osteoporosis but at this time the interrelationship between genetic factors and other determinants of bone physiology is poorly understood.*

In this connection, I recently came across a fascinating book, *Genetic Prophecy: Beyond the Double Helix*, by Dr. Zsolt Harsanyi and Richard Hutton. As the name implies, the book deals with the latest research into genetic factors that predispose a person to various diseases. Harsanyi and Hutton's basic thesis is concerned with why one person becomes ill, while another, subjected to the same environment, stays healthy. The secret, they state, "is partly contained in each individual's internal blueprint, the genes . . . disease occurs when an environmental insult meets genetic predisposition, when environmental and genetic factors come together."

The trail leading to discovery of "gene markers" which can predict susceptibility to certain diseases began in the 1930s when Peter Gorer, a researcher at Guys Hospital, London, England, came across a previously undiscovered system of mouse antigens (molecules that sit on the surface of the cells and govern the production of antibodies). Gorer named this the H2 system. The counterpart in humans is called HLA (human leucocyte antigen). And it is the presence or absence of certain of these HLAs which determines susceptibility to various diseases. The process is complicated, and true to my promise to make this a book for laypersons, I will not explore it further. Suffice it to say that today HLA markers are accepted as genetic indicators for more than 80 diseases ranging from allergies to cardiovascular disorders, to certain cancers, and more are being discovered every year.

Harsanyi and Hutton predict that in the not-too-distant future a relatively simple blood analysis may be available to test for susceptibility to a wide variety of diseases. While they don't mention osteoporosis, given the evidence of genetic involvement already documented, it is possible that HLA markers or other laboratory tests could become a factor in determining who is at risk for osteoporosis.

OSTEOPOROSIS AND OTHER DISEASES

"Chronic illness of almost any kind can lead to osteopenia, with malnutrition and disuse the major contributing factors," states Dr. Kaplan. In addition, there are several specific diseases associated with bone loss. Those mentioned most frequently in the literature are endocrine diseases, bone marrow disorders, such as myeloma or leukemia, and diabetes of long standing (rare).

For example, Dr. Kaplan writes, "Endocrine abnormalities may cause osteoporosis and should be investigated in any young or middle-aged person with osteopenia. Numerous hormones affect skeletal remodelling and hence, skeletal mass." Some of the more common endocrine disorders Dr. Kaplan cites are:

Hypogonadism or under-activity of the ovaries or testes: we have already referred to this in connection with loss of estrogen in post-menopausal women.

Hyperthyroidism or over-activity of the thyroid gland: "whether caused by glandular hyperactivity or secondary to overzealous replacement therapy . . . increases bone turnover and remodelling. . . . The clinician should check for symptoms and signs of hyperthyroidism in osteopenic patients, especially in those on long-term thyroid replacement therapy."

Hyperparathyroidism or over-activity of the parathyroid gland: "also increases bone turnover and remodelling, causing a net increase in bone resorption . . . resulting from the hypercalcemic effect of increased PTH (parathyroid hormone) secretion."

Hyperadrenalism or chronic glucocorticoid excess: "leads to a refractory state of decreased bone mass, resulting from increased bone resorption."

Although the percentage of osteoporosis attributable to these diseases and disorders is minimal, I mention them because they must be identified and/or ruled out before treatment for the more common "senile" or "post-menopausal" osteoporosis begins.

Finally, those under medication should also be aware that prolonged use of certain prescription and non-prescription drugs can affect calcium metabolism and/or bone formation and resorption. Following is a list of the more common ones with source of information in brackets.

Heparin (for anti-coagulation) (Kaplan)
Thyroid supplement (Thyroxin, Synthroid) (Kaplan)
Cortisone (Kaplan)
Certain antacids containing aluminum hydroxide (Dr. Karl Insogna, University of Rochester Medical School).

POSSIBLE CAUSES IN MY CASE

It is evident that "idiopathic" osteoporosis, as it is sometimes called, which strikes from one-quarter to one-third of post-menopausal women, may be attributable to any one, or to a combination of, causes. It would be logical to assume that those most at risk would be women whose history and lifestyle combine the highest number of risk factors.

In response to the "why me?" syndrome, I have often gone over the possible factors that could have been at work in my own case; recounting these may be helpful, at least in a speculative sense.

GENETIC

It is quite possible that a genetic factor was involved. While none of my immediate forebears was diagnosed as osteoporotic, my mother and several aunts developed the characteristic dowager's hump. And my mother had episodes of undiagnosed back ailments for many years.

PHYSICAL CHARACTERISTICS

I have been a relative lightweight all my life (5 ft. 3 in., 120 lbs. [1.6m/54 kg], prior to onset of osteoporosis). I have what in lay terms would be called a fine bone structure, so that I would not have had any excess of bone mass to begin with, and I also have the fair hair and complexion prevalent among osteoporotics.

DIET AND EXERCISE

While my lifestyle over the years should not have put me at risk in these categories, for some six months prior to the onset of acute osteoporotic symptoms my normally healthy regimen changed drastically.

A broken wrist with complications led to my wearing a heavier than normal cast for two months. During this period I spent an inordinate amount of time in a supine position, book in hand. Also at this time, and for some months thereafter, various complications in the lives of my grown children sent me into a psychological tailspin. This combination of negative circumstances made life chaotic, and I suffered acutely from stress and lack of sleep for some months. During this period I completely neglected my exercise program and paid scant attention to diet.

Whether such a brief let-up in a normally healthy lifestyle could have had an effect on calcium absorption or bone mass is difficult to say. My own feeling is that it may well have accelerated an already insidious process.

ENDOCRINE DISORDERS AND DRUG-RELATED CAUSES

For 18 years prior to the diagnosis of osteoporosis I had been taking, under prescription, 0.4 mg daily of Thyroxin to compensate for an under-active thyroid gland. When various laboratory tests confirmed the diagnosis of osteoporosis, the internist immediately began to cut the thyroid supplement. In two months he had me down to 0.1 mg a day. Now, some six years later, I am still on this moderate dosage (one-quarter of the amount I had taken for 18 years) and suffer no symptoms of thyroid hormone deficiency. I am convinced that having taken an excessive amount of thyroid supplement over such a prolonged period was, at the very least, a contributing factor to my condition.

To sum up, while no one specific cause of osteoporosis has been determined, it would be wise for women, young and old alike, to examine their possible risk factors and take appropriate defensive measures. After all, better to bar the door on the bone robber than to try and catch him after the damage has been done!

EFFECTS OF OSTEOPOROSIS

Many of these have already been described in Chapter 1. The most serious effect is the weakening of the bone structure to such an extent that fractures occur with a minimum of trauma. Some patients have reported ribs broken merely by the force of a sneeze. Bones particularly at risk are the vertebrae, the neck of the femur (hip bone), and the distal radius (wrist).

While fractures of the wrist usually heal with no lasting disability, hip fractures are, of course, much more serious. In the case of the very elderly who are most at risk, a hip fracture can be truly devastating. In fact, reports Dr. Joan Harrison, 12 per cent of elderly patients die as a direct or indirect result of hip fracture.

But since the majority of osteoporotics will be most affected by stress or crush fracturing of one or several vertebrae, let's examine this aspect more closely. Depending on the number and location of such damaged vertebrae, the patient may suffer severe pain and disability, or she may not even be aware that such a fracture has occurred. In extreme cases, as noted in Chapter 1, the effect can be totally incapacitating.

The upper spine may take on a noticeable curvature, the beginning of the dreaded dowager's hump. Depending on the number of collapsed vertebrae, the patient may lose up to several inches in height which results in a drastic structural realignment highlighted by a protruding abdomen and a walking stance both awkward and painful.

The psychological aspects of this condition, as related to my own case, have been detailed in Chapter 1.

The physical pain associated with vertebral damage and the ensuing height loss involves a change in musculature. In order to better understand this aspect, one must know the fundamentals of back anatomy.

FUNDAMENTALS OF BACK ANATOMY

There are four regions of the spine:

1. Cervical (neck area) consists of seven vertebrae capable of great motion.
2. Thoracic or dorsal (mid-back) has 12 vertebrae with special attachments for the ribs. This area of the spine is less mobile.
3. Lumbar (lower back) has five large vertebrae which bear the brunt of the weight of the upper body.
4. Sacrum and coccyx region: A broad triangular structure (the sacrum) is attached at the top to the lumbar region and on the sides to the pelvis. The coccyx is the collection of a few small bones at the end of the sacrum, commonly referred to as the tail bone.

Each vertebra is joined to the next by a capsule of layered ligament and other tissue that is roughly flat and circular in shape— the infamous disc which is blamed for a plethora of back problems.

The *pelvis*, the floor on which the lower internal organs rest, is composed of three bones—the sacrum and two ilia. The juncture of these is the sacroiliac joint. On either side of the pelvis are the sockets into which the ball-like ends of the thighbones fit to form the hip joints. The motion thus provided enables you to walk, run, climb, stoop, squat, sit, etc.

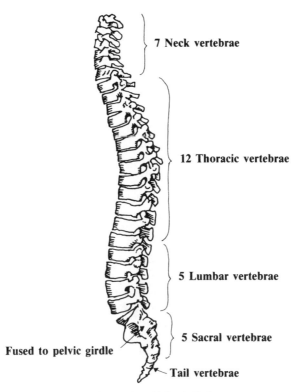

7 Neck vertebrae

12 Thoracic vertebrae

5 Lumbar vertebrae

5 Sacral vertebrae

Fused to pelvic girdle

Tail vertebrae

Figure 1a. Spinal Column

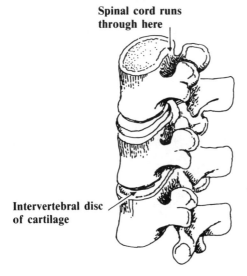

Spinal cord runs
through here

Intervertebral disc
of cartilage

Figure 1b. Lumbar Vertebrae

This is a very cursory outline of the bony spinal structure. But in order to understand clearly the effects of the collapsed vertebrae of osteoporosis, we must also have a rudimentary knowledge of the muscles, ligaments, and tendons attached to the spinal column—the binding, as it were, that holds the spinal structure in place.

Ligaments are dense, tough strands of tissue which attach one bone to another. *Tendons* are similar in structure to ligaments, but differ in function. They attach muscles to bones. *Muscles* are composed of contractible fibres which respond to nerve impulses. There are four general muscle groups which affect the back:

1. the abdominal muscles which supply frontal support;
2. the extensor muscles which hold the rear frame of the torso erect;
3. the lateral muscles which provide lateral support and sideways motion;
4. the hip muscles which, because of their relationship to the pelvis, also affect the spine.

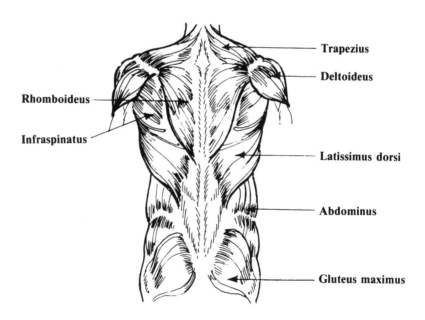

Figure 2. Muscles Supporting the Back

All these sets of muscles work together for the proper functioning of your back. To get an idea of how important the interaction of these structures is, we might compare the whole to a tent with centre pole (spine) and guy-ropes (ligaments, tendons, muscles). Now if any of the guy-ropes are weak, obviously there is going to be more stress on the centre pole. And conversely, if the centre pole is weak, or telescoped, as in the case of collapsed vertebrae, the guy-ropes will sag.

This is exactly what happens when the osteoporotic patient suddenly loses several inches in height. The guy-ropes (musculature) become slack. Their efforts to re-adjust and the resultant disturbance of nerve endings cause the excruciating pain associated with *muscle spasm*.

I wish there were a more evil-sounding term for this effect. "Spasm" sounds so innocuous, so fleeting. But as anyone who has experienced the phenomenon will know, muscle spasm is anything but innocuous and far from fleeting. As with any pain, that associated with muscle spasm originates in the nervous system. For example, if you put your finger on a hot stove a nerve impulse to the brain stimulates an answering impulse which makes you remove your finger from the stove in a fraction of a second. But when the cause of the pain is constant within your body, you cannot lift the affected part from the source. Nevertheless, the nerve message is telling the muscles to recoil and this causes muscle spasm.

From the foregoing, it is evident that keeping the musculature supporting the spine in top shape is a vital ingredient in combatting back pain. This is particularly true if you have suffered the compacting of vertebrae common to osteoporotics. Let me quote Dr. Leon Root, an orthopedic specialist, in this regard:

Although back problems caused by the aging process are often irreversible, they need not be a constant source of pain or disability. I have had many patients in their seventies and eighties who, although their spines showed the same deterioration as those of other older people, had very little in the way of back problems. These patients are invariably the ones who have, throughout their lives, taken care of the supporting structures of their backs, even strengthened them, so

that their supporting structures, especially their muscles, were able to take up the work that their spines . . . were no longer able to do.
(*Oh, My Aching Back.* David McKay, N.Y. 1973, p. 80).

SYMPTOMS OF OSTEOPOROSIS

The main obstacle to early diagnosis and treatment of osteoporosis is the fact that detectable symptoms do not appear until the disease is well advanced. Up to 30 per cent of bone mass may be lost before the deficiency shows up on routine X-rays. By that time, the bone robber has been at work for many years.

Usually the first symptoms will manifest themselves in the form of acute pain in the mid- to low-back region. This pain may occur even while at rest or during routine daily activity, or it may be traceable to some particular strain on the spinal area. In either case, it is likely due to a compression fracture of one or more vertebrae. For this reason, it is important that persistent, even mild, back pain be reported to your doctor and, particularly if you are a post-menopausal woman, that the possibility of osteoporosis be taken into account.

Other more dramatic symptoms are fractures of rib, hip, or wrist, or a combination of these, having occurred without definitely traceable traumatic cause. Height loss could be another indication of osteopenia. You should keep track of your height and report any dramatic loss to your doctor. Because compression fractures of vertebrae do not always cause undue pain, height loss may be the first symptom you notice. There may also be a rounding of the shoulders if affected vertebrae are in the upper-back region.

Dental X-rays may offer another clue. In some cases bone loss in the jaw can be an early symptom. You might ask your dentist whether routine X-rays reveal any loss of density in the jawbone.

Unfortunately, these often nebulous factors may be the only indication you have that the bone robber has invaded your premises. It is to be hoped that the more accurate methods of measuring bone mass used in large research hospitals (see Chapter 3) will become more available nationwide, thus permitting easier screening of patients at risk from osteoporosis. In fact, there is evidence that this is happening, but in the meantime it is up to each individual to be on the alert and, above all, to look to her defences.

Chapter 3
Managing
the Beast

This chapter deals with what you and your doctor, working together, can do with regard to preventive measures, earlier diagnosis, and treatment of osteoporosis. Unfortunately, the most promising treatment therapies are barely past the experimental stages, but research continues on a number of fronts. Later in the chapter we'll outline some of the more promising projects and their results to date. But first, let's look at more widely accepted procedures.

DOCTOR RESPONSIBILITY

The first responsibility of the physician is, of course, to diagnose the condition. Unfortunately, many centres in North America do not have specialists trained in metabolic bone disease and bone pathology, and many general practitioners are still not fully cognizant of the danger of osteoporosis. It would be helpful if all doctors were concerned with educating their post-menopausal patients in this regard, and in having them take precautionary measures in the following categories.

DIET

Since osteoporosis is a condition which affects one in four post-menopausal women (some sources say one in three), general practitioners should be on the lookout for early symptoms. While doctors may be wary of frightening their patients unnecessarily, they could question the dietary habits of post-menopausal women, particularly with regard to calcium intake, without causing undue alarm.

EXERCISE

Doctors may well feel that this is the patient's own responsibility. Most women, however, aren't aware of the relationship between exercise and retention of bone mass. It would seem a simple matter for doctors to stress the importance of adequate exercise, even perhaps recommending a specific program for post-menopausal patients.

HEIGHT LOSS

I believe every annual checkup should include measurement of height as well as of weight. Any reduction in height greater than that attributable to normal aging would sound a red alert for osteoporosis. I realize that by the time height loss is evident, crush fractures will have already occurred. Since there can be such vertebral fractures with little or no pain, however, it is entirely possible that height loss may be the first measurable symptom of osteoporosis.

TREATMENT

The other major doctor responsibility is, of course, the treatment and handling of the condition once it has been diagnosed. Since opinions within the medical profession vary widely as to the most effective medications, I will not presume to offer advice in this regard. I have already mentioned (Chapter 1) the regimen I was on, but I freely admit that some of these medications, particularly sodium fluoride, are still at the clinical investigation stage, and are not, therefore, widely available. The use of estrogen and vitamin D supplements are also somewhat controversial.

Despite differing opinions about these more radical therapies, there now seems to be a consensus among doctors on the need for adequate calcium intake throughout life. Some doctors are skeptical, however, about the efficacy of calcium supplementation alone in treating established osteoporosis. A complete dietary analysis of osteoporotic patients would appear reasonable, however, to enable the physician to prescribe the correct amount of calcium supplement should it be necessary to do so.

We have already mentioned the exercise factor with reference to prevention of osteoporosis. Once the condition has been diagnosed, however, it is even more essential that a proper exercise program be undertaken. A detailed program might be prescribed by the doctor directly or he might refer the patient to a physiotherapist who is thoroughly acquainted with the special needs of osteoporotics. I don't think it's enough for the doctor to say "you must walk a lot" or "you must see that you get adequate exercise." Patients may soon forget such vague advice, or be unsure just what constitutes "adequate exercise." If a specific program were prescribed by a competent physiotherapist, the patient would be more likely to take it seriously.

I think doctors also have a responsibility to help their osteoporotic patients deal with the physical and psychological aspects of any dramatic height loss.

Let's look first at the physical aspects. Compression of abdominal organs can lead to an almost constant bloated feeling, so that eating becomes a duty rather than a pleasure. I eventually discovered that eating smaller meals at more frequent intervals helped considerably. Doctors should, I feel, discuss this phenomenon with their patients.

Then there is the unbalancing effect of the altered skeletal structure. I felt as though I had to learn to walk all over again, and, even now, I'm conscious of a somewhat awkward gait. When I first began to walk long distances I experienced considerable pain in the left thigh. One day, when walking on a hillside, I discovered that this pain went away when the left leg was on a higher incline than the right. I reported this to my doctor, who prescribed specially molded inserts for my shoes, the left one slightly higher at the heel. These helped considerably, and I only wished I'd had them from the beginning.

This experience led me to conclude that anyone who has suffered drastic skeletal alteration should be referred to an orthopedic specialist. It would seem essential that accurate measurements be taken and professional advice offered on handling the condition.

Professional advice would also be helpful in dealing with the psychological aspects of acute osteoporosis. I strongly recommend that osteoporotic patients be referred to psychologists, where possible. I know I would have appreciated talking to someone who understood the traumatic psychological implications of having suddenly lost four inches (10 cm) in height, gained a like number around the middle, and assumed a bent-over posture more suitable to a woman of 90 than to one in her mid-50s. I was lucky in that I had a supportive family who helped me "muddle through" the psychological trauma. But many women have to cope on their own and would greatly benefit from an understanding listener.

PATIENT RESPONSIBILITY

LIFESTYLE

The first and foremost patient responsibility is maintaining a line of defence. It is not my purpose to create unnecessary fear of osteoporosis or to encourage women to run to their doctors with imagined symptoms. I merely want to alert them to the danger so that they can be on guard. It is relatively simple to ensure that your diet contains adequate calcium, that you get some form of regular exercise, and that you avoid or, at the very least, reduce alcohol and tobacco consumption. While these measures won't guarantee immunity from osteoporosis, they could go a long way towards minimizing the effect.

DRUGS

It is also a good idea to be alert to the side effects of any medications you take regularly. In Chapter 2, I have listed some prescription and non-prescription drugs which can interfere with calcium absorption and/or increase calcium excretion. If you are on any of these medications, you may wish to discuss possible side effects with your doctor. Reduced dosage or substitute medication may be possibilities.

UNDIAGNOSED BACK PAIN

If you are in the "high risk" category for osteoporosis you should be doubly alert if your back begins to act up. If you aren't responding to conventional treatment, insist on an X-ray. I realize that physicians are loathe to prescribe X-rays unnecessarily, but if there is cause to suspect osteoporosis, the sooner you know, the better. While it is true that up to 30 per cent of bone mass may be lost before it is discernible on routine X-ray, it is entirely possible to reach this condition without having experienced previous noticeable symptoms.

CURRENT RESEARCH

Perhaps the most optimistic note for osteoporotic patients is the increasing awareness of the condition among both doctors and laypersons. During the past few years, symposia have been held at several major centres. Members of the Energy and Chemical Workers Union across Canada pledged $750,000 to support osteoporosis research. Projects aimed at finding better diagnostic and treatment methods are burgeoning in the United States as well, and throughout the western hemisphere. Later in this chapter we'll examine a few such projects.

Because treatment and diagnosis of osteoporosis requires an accurate method of measuring bone mass and calcium loss, we must begin with a summary of the more sophisticated methods of making such measurements.

MEASUREMENT OF BONE LOSS

Since there will be reference to cortical and trabecular bone in several of the methods outlined below, a brief definition of these terms is in order.

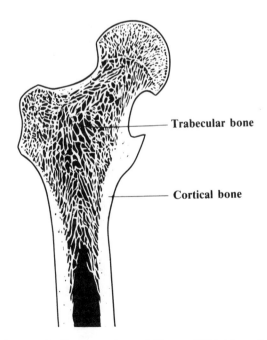

Figure 3. Cross-section of Femur (Thighbone)

39

Cortical bone is relatively dense, while trabecular bone is more porous, resembling a honeycomb with its lace-like structure. All bones are composed of both types, trabecular bone nearest the centre, enclosed by the more solid cortical bone. Parts of the skeleton differ, however, in the relative amounts of each type of bone they contain. The long bones of the extremities are predominantly cortical, while the vertebrae are composed almost entirely of trabecular bone with a thin protective coating of cortical. There is also a higher proportion of trabecular bone in the ends of the long bones than along their length.

The following is a brief description of the methods most commonly used to measure bone mass.

X-ray As stated previously, ordinary X-rays are not very helpful in early diagnosis of osteoporosis since decreased bone mass may not be evident until up to 30 per cent has been lost. X-rays are valuable, however, in detecting crush fractures, in determining the degree of osteoporotic damage in severe cases, and possibly in distinguishing such damage from other causes of back pain.

Radiogrammetry This method involves X-raying the second metacarpal (middle finger between wrist and knuckles) in order to estimate the cortical thickness. While it is easy to perform and can be repeated frequently, the method is not sensitive enough to serve as a screening tool for osteoporosis. Since it measures only cortical bone, it is of no use in assessing spinal (trabecular) bone loss.

Radiographic Photodensitometry This method involves the bones of the middle segment of the fingers (phalanges). A piece of aluminum alloy is placed next to the hand when the X-ray is taken. Afterwards a computer scanner compares the density of the bone with the known density of the aluminum alloy. Here again the disadvantage is that radiographic photodensitometry cannot be used to measure the trabecular bone of the spine. Also, the technique involves equipment that is not available at all hospitals.

Single-photon Absorptiometry In this method the absorption of a photon beam is measured as it passes through bone tissue. The difference in photon absorption in bone and in soft tissue allows measurement of the mineral content in the extremities or long bones where cortical bone is predominant. It is not, however, effective for measuring bone mass in the predominantly trabecular bone of the spinal column. Measurements with single-photon absorptiometry are usually taken in the radius (forearm).

Dual-photon Absorptiometry This is an improvement on single-photon absorptiometry in that it allows measurement of the axial skeleton (spine). It involves use of a radioactive isotope which emits photons at two different energy levels, allowing differentiation of fat and soft tissue from bone. Since it permits measurement of bone mass in the spinal area, this technique is particularly applicable to osteoporotics. As with single-photon absorptiometry, radiation is minimal. The main disadvantages are the expense and the relative unavailability of the required apparatus.

Quantitative Computed Tomography (C.T. Scan) Dr. Morris Notelovitz, Professor of Obstetrics and Gynecology at the University of Florida College of Medicine, terms the C.T. scan "the most accurate method of determining early bone loss in the spine." (*Stand Tall! Every Woman's Guide To Preventing Osteoporosis*, p. 86) And M. Banna, Associate Professor of Neuroradiology, McMaster University, Hamilton, Ontario, states: "The device has been universally acclaimed as second in importance only to Roentgen's discovery of X-rays in 1895." The C.T. scanner provides a view of a series of transverse slices of the area being X-rayed. It reflects the basic elements present within or between cells. Bone contains a lot of calcium which absorbs more radiation and appears white on the C.T. image.

Here again the disadvantage of the C.T. scanner is its expense and relative unavailability for use in early detection of bone loss or for routine follow-up of osteoporotic patients. The relatively high radiation dose involved in a body scan is also a negative factor.

Dr. T. N. Hangartner, formerly of the Department of Applied Sciences in Medicine, University of Alberta, and his colleague Dr. T. R. Overton, however, have modified a special purpose C.T. scanner with a radioisotope photon source to provide sensitive high-precision measurements of both cortical and trabecular bone. Measurements with this special purpose scanner are taken at the distal end of the radius.

Neutron Activation Analysis In this method the skeleton is exposed to a flux of high-energy neutrons. This makes the calcium content of the bones radioactive. The radioactivity is then measured by its gamma ray emission, providing an accurate measurement of bone mineral mass. Comments Dr. Joan Harrison, "Using neutron activation analysis it is possible to detect the loss of bone mass and consequently to determine the increased risk of osteoporotic fractures." Dr. Harrison emphasizes the importance of measuring skeletal changes in the central rather than the peripheral skeleton, since bones of the trunk and hips are most at risk from fracture.

Once again, however, this technique is available only in research centres, which precludes its use as a general screening device or as a universal method of measuring changes in the bone mass of osteoporotic patients.

Transiliac Bone Biopsy This technique involves taking a tiny plug of bone from the hip for analysis. Tetracycline is given orally for three days before the biopsy. This serves as a time-spaced fluorescent marker to allow measurement of bone formation. The extraction of the bone plug is done with a special bone biopsy needle. Only local anaesthetic is used. Usually it is an out-patient procedure with ambulation permitted the same day.

While this method would seem to be less expensive and more widely available than some of the others, it is not suitable for routine screening purposes. It can, however, be useful for patient follow-up.

These are the eight methods of measuring bone mass most frequently mentioned in the literature. I must, however, include one other very recent innovation.

The Osteoquant A publication of the Miami Valley Hospital, Dayton, Ohio, *Insider*, reports in a bulletin entitled "Biomedical Imaging Director Invents Device to Detect Osteoporosis" (April 8, 1988) on a further breakthrough by Dr. Hangartner, now a director of the Biomedical Imaging Laboratory of Miami Valley Hospital and Wright State University.

After 12 years of research Dr. Hangartner has developed the Osteoquant, described in the bulletin as:

> *. . . a device capable of measuring bone loss to 0.5 per-*
> *cent precision compared to the three percent associated*
> *with the C.T. scan.*
>
> *Hangartner's Osteoquant is the only one of its kind*
> *in the U.S., and one of only three in the world. It pro-*
> *duces a three-dimensional representation of the bone*
> *by taking X-ray pictures at 128 different angles. All*
> *this is done in little over a minute.*
>
> *The Osteoquant, which resembles a large metal*
> *donut, uses a complex mathematical formula to pro-*
> *duce the image of the bone that is then reflected on*
> *a television screen. After the patient inserts either an*
> *arm or a leg through the hole in the machine, five to*
> *ten images of the bone appear on the screen.*

This would appear to be a dramatic breakthrough, but, again, availability is a problem.

While the highly sophisticated methods of bone mass measurement are becoming increasingly available, many hospitals still lack the necessary equipment. This, I believe, is a major stumbling block to earlier diagnosis and more successful treatment of osteoporosis. I have personally felt frustrated by the situation, since I would dearly love to know to what extent the tremendous improvement in my condition is due to increase in bone mass (if any) and to what extent to other factors such as increased muscular fitness.

I had three series of back and hip X-rays during the two or three years following the onset of osteoporotic symptoms. These showed no further deterioration, nor any perceptible increase in bone mass. This frustrating uncertainty is, I imagine, shared by most osteoporotic patients, particularly those who live outside major population centres where hospitals' diagnostic facilities may be limited.

BLOOD AND URINE TESTS AS A DIAGNOSTIC TOOL

With regard to earlier diagnosis of osteoporosis and assessment of at-risk patients, readers might wonder why blood and/or urine tests could not be used to indicate loss of calcium. Unfortunately, there is no simple blood test for calcium content which would indicate bone mineral deterioration. A blood test for calcium can appear normal even when large amounts have been lost from the bone. For screening patients already known to have lost bone mass, blood tests are useful, however, because they help the clinician to distinguish bone loss due to osteoporosis from that due to other causes. Similarly, urine tests are not generally considered helpful in early diagnosis because severely osteoporotic patients may show normal amounts of calcium in the urine.

There is hope on the horizon. Dr. Claus Christiansen, Chairman of the Department of Clinical Chemistry at Glostrup Hospital, University of Copenhagen, heads a team doing research in this field. At a 1984 meeting of the Toronto Calcium and Bone Club, Dr. Christiansen reported that his team had discovered that post-menopausal women at risk of developing osteoporosis may be detected by a blood test and fasting urine sample corrected for creatinine. Since the calcium in the fasting urine sample would come only from the bones, it was reasoned that this would be an indication of bone turnover.

A later report on the studies at Glostrup was published in *The Lancet* (May 16, 1987) under the title, "Prediction of Rapid Bone Loss in Postmenopausal Women." Dr. Christiansen, B. J. Riis, and P. Rødbro measured loss of bone mass in 178 women in the early post-menopausal period, using the photon absorptiometry method, every three months for two years. The results were compared with those of a single determination of body fat mass, urinary calcium and hydroxyproline, and serum alkaline phosphatase carried out at the first examination.

Christiansen and his associates found that the fast bone mass losers (as measured by photon absorptiometry) were characterized by higher fasting urinary hydroxyproline and calcium levels, lower serum oestrone and oestradiol levels, and lower body weight than the slow losers. Thus, the report concludes, "with only one blood sample and one urine sample (plus measurement of height and weight), the majority (79%) of post-menopausal women at risk of osteoporosis can be identified at reasonable cost."

While these results from Glostrup are indeed encouraging with regard to earlier screening of at-risk patients, universally available means of accurately measuring bone mass remain elusive.

Research on other fronts, however, appears promising. Many projects, underway in various parts of the world, are researching the efficacy of different treatment methods in arresting or reversing bone loss. There is not enough space to describe even a fraction of them in detail. A cursory examination of a few projects involving more controversial current therapies is in order, however. Here is a random sample.

SODIUM FLUORIDE

One of the most prominent projects in Canada has been in progress for a number of years at the University of Toronto's Bone and Mineral Metabolism Unit headed by Dr. Joan Harrison.

Thirty-two patients with post-menopausal osteoporosis were followed for periods of three years or more to assess the effects of treatment on bone mineral mass. Measurements were done by neutron activation analysis. Serum fluoride concentrations were also measured, and bone biopsies carried out in some cases.

The treatment consisted of various combinations of NaF (sodium fluoride), 25 mg, twice daily; calcium, 1 g a day; vitamin D_2, 50,000 IU, twice weekly; and estrogen, 0.625 mg a day. NaF was always given in combination with calcium and vitamin D_2. Seven patients received estrogen in addition to NaF and nine received NaF without estrogen.

For eight of these latter 16 patients there was no evidence of adequate fluoride retention. The eight patients adequately treated with NaF, however, demonstrated on average a 13 per cent increase in bone mineral mass. This sounds promising indeed, but we must remember that this study involved a small number of patients. And as Dr. Harrison points out, there are problems to be resolved with sodium fluoride treatment. She mentions two in particular: "why some subjects need much higher doses of fluoride than others in order to stimulate bone growth"; and "how to prevent adverse reactions, gastrointestinal irritation and bone pain and tenderness."

In a paper presented to the International Symposium on Osteoporosis, Denmark, in 1987, Harrison and her associates report some success with a coated fluoride preparation to reduce or eliminate gastrointestinal symptoms. However, this treatment is not yet available for general use.

Later studies by Dr. Harrison and associates examined the relationship between fluoride effects on bone histology (tissue structure), bone mass, and bone strength. This project sought a method to assess, at an earlier stage, the efficacy of fluoride treatment in individual patients, and to ascertain the optimal dosage, which can vary from patient to patient.

Reports on these studies are given in three recent publications: (1) *Bone and Mineral 1* (1986); (2) a brief summary of a presentation at the International Symposium on Osteoporosis, Denmark, 1987; and (3) *Journal of Bone and Mineral Research* (Vol. 3, No. 2, 1988). These reports are too technical for my purposes but are listed in the Bibliography for the benefit of professionals who might be interested.

The last-mentioned report concludes: "We consider the histological assessment on biopsy, taken within the initial two years of treatment, as the most reliable predictor of satisfactory fluoride effects on bone mass, but longer follow-up of these patients is required to provide further confirmation." The paper given at the Denmark Symposium concludes: "Overall, fluoride is beneficial for the majority of osteoporotic patients."

Other researchers involved with sodium fluoride therapy include groups at the Mayo Clinic, the Henry Ford Hospital in Detroit, and a team in Lyon, France. Commenting on the work at the Mayo Clinic, Dr. Riggs stated: "the combination of calcium, fluoride and estrogen was more effective than any other combination. These results provide grounds for optimism about the efficacy of combinations of available agents with sodium fluoride for fracture prevention in post-menopausal osteoporosis."

Although not yet approved by the FDA (Food and Drug Administration) in the United States or by the HPB (Health Protection Branch) in Canada, some specialists are prescribing sodium fluoride therapy in desperate cases (mine was a prime example). And in an article published in *Practical Therapeutics* (December 1987) Drs. Mark Ziloski and Lewis B. Morrow, both on the faculty of the Medical College of Ohio, state:

> *If there are a number of vertebral compression fractures, sodium fluoride can be added. . . . Preliminary data indicate that, when used with calcium and estrogen, a daily dosage of 50 to 80 mg of sodium fluoride can lead to an increase in bone mass. . . . We recommend that patients receiving fluoride also be given 1.2 g of calcium daily.*

COHERENCE THERAPY OR ADFR (ACTIVATE, DEPRESS, FREE, REPEAT)

A study by Drs. C. Anderson, R.D.T. Cape, R. G. Crilly, A. B. Hodsman, and B.M.J. Wolfe of the University of Western Ontario involved a form of coherence therapy administered cyclically. Each cycle consisted of (a) an initial administration of two tablets of Phosphate Sandoz three times daily for three days, followed by (b) 15 days of a dose of Didronel (sodium diphosphonate) equal to 5 mg a day per kg of bodyweight, and (c) a medication-free period from day 19 to day 89 except to ensure that the diet included a minimum calcium intake of 1 g a day. Cycles were repeated at 90-day intervals with clinical examination between cycles.

All patients in the study reported improvement in their symptoms between the end of the second and the end of the third cycles. There were marked increases in their daily activities with a corresponding decrease in pain. With respect to bone density, the clinicians report "total trabecular bone volume and trabecular diameter (as measured by trans-iliac crest biopsy) increased in extent far beyond those increases reported by other therapeutic regimens attempting to restore bone mass to osteoporotic individuals, especially after six cycles of this form of therapy."

In a follow-up letter dated June 7, 1988, Dr. Anderson advises that their pilot project ended in 1987, and the results have been submitted for publication. He goes on to say that the concept has to be investigated further because various drugs (prescribed for skeletal or other conditions) interfere with it. Readers interested in further information on this study might refer to synopses of papers presented at a meeting in Aalburg, Denmark in 1987.

ESTROGEN

Dr. Heaney reports on studies done at Creighton University on the role of the deficiency of estrogen and calcium in development of a post-menopausal osteoporosis. These studies began in 1967 on a stable population of 200 women whose ages upon entering the study ranged from 36 to 45 years. They were brought into the clinic once every five years for metabolic and bone loss studies, but their diet and medical care were not interfered with.

One of the first things that became evident was the relationship between calcium balance and dietary calcium intake. It was further noted that estrogen status was related to the calcium balances of the individuals. Those who were pre-menopausal, or whose physicians had placed them on estrogen therapy, had a better calcium balance than post-menopausal women not treated with estrogen. In the women who reached menopause during the course of the study and were untreated, there was a definite deterioration in calcium balance. Dr. Heaney summarizes their findings:

We have been able to observe a linear relationship between calcium intake and calcium balance, both for the estrogen replete and the estrogen deprived women . . . women do less well in terms of calcium balance performance in the absence of estrogen. They absorb more efficiently in the presence of estrogen and urinary calcium loss is less in the presence of estrogen than in the absence of estrogen.

From a perusal of later research studies and recommended therapies, it is abundantly clear that the use of estrogen therapy has won a high degree of acceptance among the medical community. To quote two of its many advocates, Drs. Ziloski and Morrow of the Ohio Medical College:

Menopause, whether natural or surgically produced is the most important risk factor for osteoporosis. We believe that estrogen therapy is the most effective means of protecting against the rapid loss of bone that follows menopause . . . for those at high risk of osteoporosis such as slender, fair-skinned smokers with a family history of the disease, we . . . strongly recommend estrogen therapy as well as cessation of smoking.

Drs. Ziloski and Morrow go on to state that the risk of endometrial cancer is small and can be further reduced by the addition of medroxyprogesterone (10 mg a day) from day 15 to day 25 of the cycle. While the usual recommended dose of estrogen is 0.625 mg a day, the doctors state that "a dosage of only 0.3 mg of conjugated estrogens, accompanied by 1.2 g of calcium per day, may prevent osteoporosis."

They also report on a more recently developed method of estrogen administration:

> . . . the use of the estradiol transdermal system (estra-derm) which contains less estrogen and avoids the first-pass liver effect . . . is beneficial in preventing post-menopausal bone loss, and may further decrease the adverse effects of estrogen therapy. The new patches (applied externally) contain . . . estradiol and are changed every three days.

On a personal note, I might add that my latest research for this publication, conducted in the spring of 1988, so convinced me of the efficacy of estrogen therapy that I was persuaded to resume such treatment after an estrogen-free period of three years. I had been reluctant to incorporate the protective progesterone component, which had not been part of my former regimen, because progesterone is added to protect the uterine lining by inducing menstruation. After all, what woman wants to give up one of the few perks of old age? I was somewhat mollified, how-ever, when my doctor said that at my age (60) it would be neces-sary to induce menstruation only once every three or four months and that I can exercise some choice in the matter of timing.

CALCITONIN

Several sources mention recent studies relating calcitonin therapy to prevention of bone loss. In order to understand this relation-ship, one must know a little about the body's mechanism for maintaining the correct calcium balance in the blood. Although 99 per cent of the calcium in our bodies is stored in the bones, that vital 1 per cent in the bloodstream must be maintained at a constant level in order to properly regulate nerve, muscle, and cardiac functions. When the calcium level in the bloodstream drops, the parathyroid glands release a hormone commonly known as PTH (parathyroid hormone), which stimulates bone resorption, releasing the needed calcium from the bones. But should too much calcium be released into the bloodstream, it can accumulate in the arteries and soft tissues, a very dangerous situation.

Nature guards against this danger by providing a counter-balance to PTH in the hormone calcitonin, produced by the thyroid gland. Calcitonin inhibits bone resorption. The combination of PTH, calcitonin, and the active metabolite of vitamin D working together to maintain proper blood calcium levels is indeed a marvelous and delicate mechanism.

Drs. Ziloski and Morrow, referred to above, state that calcitonin-salmon has a short-term effect in decreasing calcium resorption and increasing bone density. They recommend 100 IU per day administered subcutaneously, along with calcium supplementation.

Another source, *The Lancet* (December 26, 1987), outlines a study at the University of Liège in Belgium, which had promising results with calcitonin-salmon administered by nasal spray. Similar studies are ongoing at the University of Copenhagen's Faculty of Medicine.

Although calcitonin therapy does not increase bone mass, it appears to be effective in preventing further loss in post-menopausal subjects.

CALCITRIOL AND/OR PARATHYROID HORMONE

Various researchers have investigated the use of calcitriol (the final active metabolite of vitamin D) administered with or without other agents. Prominent among these is Dr. Chris Gallagher of Creighton University, who obtained promising results combining calcitriol with a low calcium intake to avoid the complications of high blood or urine calcium. And a group in Boston had good results treating male osteoporotics with a combination of calcitriol and synthetic parathyroid hormone injections.

Dr. Robert G. Josse, at the Department of Medicine of the University of Toronto, lists among promising bone-formation-stimulating regimens synthetic parathyroid hormone (with or without calcitriol). In a recent article he states: "Substantial increases in vertebral bone density without evidence of accelerated appendicular cortical bone loss have been seen, but the data are very preliminary" ("Drug Treatment of Osteoporosis" *Drug Protocol* 1988: 3, 5).

THE EXERCISE FACTOR

Another front on which research continues is the role of exercise in maintaining bone mass. Some earlier studies in this field were reported in Chapter 2 and need not be repeated.

More recently, a paper authored by Drs. Raphael Chow, Joan Harrison, and James Dornan of the Queen Elizabeth Hospital Bone and Mineral Group, University of Toronto, was presented at the 6th International Symposium on Adapted Physical Activity, Brisbane, Australia (June 1987). Termed the PRO (Prevention and Rehabilitation of Osteoporosis) program, this Toronto clinic has as its goals:

1) To prevent bone loss, 2) to restore and maximize functional capacity of osteoporotic patients.

The program consists of four components:

1) educational seminars on various topics related to osteoporosis; 2) social function; 3) exercise class, three times per week; and 4) research on the effect of physical activities on osteoporosis.

At the time of the report there were 300 patients enrolled in the program, ranging in age from 47 to 82 years (average age 66.5). Patients undergo yearly bone mineral content measurements using either neutron activation analysis or dual-photon absorptiometry.

The exercise classes are conducted by an exercise fitness leader in the Queen Elizabeth Hospital gymnasium. The protocol consists of a 30-minute submaximal muscle-strengthening session and 30 minutes of aerobic activities.

The paper reported data on 90 patients who had been followed for two years. Fifty-three of these who exercised at least three times a week were designated as the exercise group. The remaining 37, who had opted to exercise at home but did not follow through, were classified as the non-exercise group. To quote from Dr. Chow's paper:

At the two-year follow up the exercise group, compared to the non-exercise group, had a much lower fracture occurrence, and none of the fractures occurred while performing the exercises. . . . There was a two to three-fold improvement in back pain seen in the exercise group. Sixty per cent of the patients in this group were pain free after the two year study. The severity of back pain in the non-exercise group, on the other hand, increased to moderate or severe intensity in two-thirds of the patients. . . . A questionnaire survey showed that those who exercised reported an improvement in general well-being, stamina and strength, and also an increase in self confidence in carrying out certain tasks, such as venturing outside the home during the winter months. . . . The program is now established as an out-patient ambulatory care facility of the Q.E. Hospital in Toronto.

A further report on the work of Dr. Chow and his associates relating bone mass to exercise appeared in the *British Medical Journal* (December 5, 1987). It concluded: ". . . we are therefore encouraged that . . . density measurements on the trunk, spine, and pelvis have detected a significant improvement in bone mineral mass [in the exercise group compared to the control group]."

I was indeed pleased to receive these two reports which confirm my long-held conviction as to the efficacy of exercise in improving both the physical and psychological well-being of osteoporotics.

SUMMARY OF CURRENT RESEARCH

A comprehensive paper on osteoporosis and the various therapies under study was published in *Drug Protocol* (May 1988). This report, entitled "Drug Treatment of Osteoporosis," by Dr. Josse, is one of the most readable (from a layperson's viewpoint) that I have come across.

While research on all fronts appears promising, clinicians emphasize that most of the newer therapies are still in the experimental stage and should not be employed without close monitoring.

It appears from a study of current medical publications, however, that estrogen therapy for post-menopausal at-risk women is becoming more accepted. While the combination of a minimal estrogen dosage (usually 0.625 mg a day), or the external patch system previously mentioned, and adequate calcium intake does not significantly improve bone mass, it does appear to prevent the rapid occurrence of bone loss in the decade following menopause.

While there is a slightly increased risk of endometrial cancer (cancer of the uterus) with estrogen therapy, one clinician points out that the usually recommended supplement is only one-third the amount contained in low dose oral contraceptives. To counteract this minimal risk, however, most doctors recommend inclusion of the progesterone cycle to protect the uterus (see personal note above). Estrogen therapy is contraindicated for women who have had cancer of the breast, uterus, or reproductive tract. Patients with a history of blood clotting disorders, high blood pressure, or heart disease should also be wary.

The use of sodium fluoride therapy is much more controversial. In some cases it has been proven to actually increase bone mass, although the bone formed in this way may be weaker than normal bone. Other patients are unable to tolerate fluoride at all. So far researchers are not recommending it for general use, and it has not yet been approved by the FDA or the HPB. Results in experimental studies are certainly promising, however, and some doctors are prescribing fluoride for severely osteoporotic patients.

The use of calcitonin, either by subcutaneous administration or as a nasal spray, is still regarded as experimental and is not in general use. Research in this area continues.

To conclude on a hopeful note, one could say that osteoporosis should no longer be looked on as an inevitable consequence of aging. Preventive measures can be taken, for example, ensuring an adequate calcium intake throughout life, combined with a daily exercise regimen and minimal or zero consumption of alcohol and tobacco. While these measures don't guarantee immunity, they do constitute a line of defence which, at the very least, should reduce the incidence and severity of the condition.

Post-menopausal at-risk women also have the option of discussing with their physicians the possibility of calcium and estrogen therapy as a preventive measure. And, if in spite of all precautions osteoporosis does strike, there is still hope that certain combinations of drugs may effect an improvement in bone mass or, at the very least, arrest the deterioration.

Chapter 4
Tips
on Coping

Let's suppose that in spite of all precautions, you have been diagnosed as osteoporotic. Whether or not you are in hospital, if your case is severe, you may be suffering acute back pain with attendant loss of mobility. The first thing to realize is that this is not a permanent situation. You can and will improve with time, patience, and perseverance. If you can adopt a positive attitude (not easy, I realize, under the circumstances), you will have leaped the first major hurdle on the road to recovery.

The first purpose of this book is to help you avoid the agony of uncertainty that I endured for some months when improvement seemed negligible. The second purpose is to help you to better cope with your disability by employing the gadgets and gimmicks that helped me so much. There are also practical steps you can take to help yourself. Let's begin with the basics—aids to, and methods for, more comfortable lying, sleeping, standing and walking, and sitting.

LYING

The most pressing problem for any back pain sufferer is how to be comfortable in bed, and how to get up and down with a minimum of pain. The bed itself should have a firm, but not rock-hard, mattress. You may want to insert a board between box-spring and mattress for added support.

I found the most comfortable lying position was flat on my back with a bolster under the knees. (Mine is a rolled up foam, 20 inches [50 cm] long and 12 inches [30 cm] in diameter, fastened with two straps and enclosed in a pillow case.) With this bolster under my knees and a couple of pillows under my head (the upper one a small feather pillow which adjusts comfortably to the contours of the neck), I found I could read in bed without strain on any part of the anatomy.

But getting into that comfortable position was something else. After much suffering and experimenting with different ways of getting in and out of bed, I learned this simple trick from the home therapist.

a. Sit on the side of the bed.
b. Lift bent knees onto the bed, and at the same time, using your arms for support, lower the upper body. You are now lying on your side with knees bent. Because adjusting from one position to another is so painful, try to land where you want to be, e.g., with your head centred on the pillow.
c. Now, still with knees bent, extend your arms and "log-roll" onto your back. This manoeuvre is key to minimizing the pain of turning from side to back or from side to side. The object is to turn the whole body in one motion so that you avoid twisting your back. Many of the tricks involved in managing back pain entail keeping the "building block" vertebrae aligned in as straight a row as possible.

To get out of bed, you reverse the above procedure—lying on your side, knees bent, use your arms to push up to sitting position, at the same time lowering your feet to the floor. You are now sitting on the edge of the bed. To stand up, place your hands on the bed behind you and push up to standing position, again taking the strain of rising off the impaired back.

SLEEPING POSITION

Probably the best position for sleeping is on your back with a small pliable pillow for your head and a bolster under your knees. I, for one, however, have great difficulty sleeping on my back, so I opted for the next best alternative. This involves lying on your side, knees bent, with a thin pliable pillow under your head, another between your knees, and one tucked firmly in at your back. The object of all these pillows is to ensure that your spinal column maintains as straight an alignment as possible. Anything remotely resembling sleeping on the stomach is a no-no for back patients.

a.

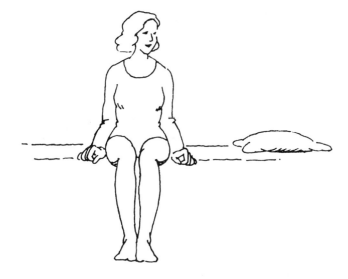

b.

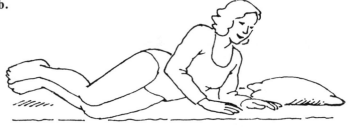

c.

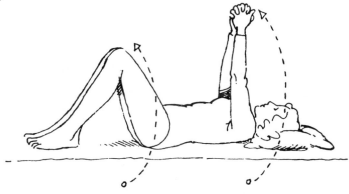

Figure 4. Towards a Comfortable Lying Position

STANDING AND WALKING

If you are an osteoporotic patient suffering acute back pain, you will be faced with the "Catch-22" situation of requiring bed rest for your ailing back, coupled with the need to walk as much as possible to prevent further bone loss. As stated earlier, I worked out a compromise, alternating periods of bed rest with route marches through the house and, at least once a day, outside.

The therapist advocated adopting the pelvic tilt (see Chapter 6) when standing or walking. At first I found this difficult, but I did try to keep my stomach tucked in and to stand as straight as possible under the circumstances. Don't be discouraged if you are quite stooped to begin with. While there is no way you can counteract the spinal damage itself, you'll find that as you work at strengthening the supporting muscles, you'll be able to straighten up considerably.

When standing for any length of time it is good to rest one foot on a low stool. This flattens the small of the back and is more comfortable than keeping both feet on the ground. I keep a sturdy metal stool handy in the kitchen for this one-foot-raised routine, and I also stand on it to reach things in high cupboards. If you're going to use your stool for this latter purpose, be sure it is firm and solidly constructed.

Actually, I find that when doing certain tasks of relatively short duration, such as mixing cookie dough or making a sandwich, it's even more comfortable to stand with one foot on a kitchen chair. But you'll still need that low stool for many household chores.

You'll likely need a walking cane, too. Choose a sturdy one of comfortable height with a good rubber tip. Because your newly-aligned spinal column is apt to make you feel insecure, the cane is important for psychological as well as for physical support. Don't be ashamed to use it for as long as necessary. I don't need my cane any longer in good weather, but still never venture forth without it if there's the least chance of encountering icy conditions.

In 1985, in Britain, I purchased an ingenious walking-stick seat. It isn't the traditional one-pronged shooting stick, but has a two-legged aluminum frame with a narrow canvas strip stretched between. Folded up it is a light-weight walking stick; unfolded, a comfortable seat.

During our rambles over hill and dale in Europe, this gadget was invaluable, as it enabled me to grab a few minutes' rest from time to time, thereby greatly extending the distance I was able to cover. It also came in handy in art galleries and museums as, in addition to the seat, it has a crossbar some six inches (15 cm) from the ground that enabled me to assume the one-foot-elevated stance when examining paintings or reading the inevitably lengthy explanations of museum items.

I bought this seat stick at a British National Trust store and am not sure whether a similar product is available in North America. If you can find such an item, I would highly recommend it.

SITTING

Though therapists caution against sitting in the acute phase of back disability, it is impossible to avoid doing so entirely. The first "gadget" I acquired on leaving hospital was a comfortable, upright, platform rocker with arms, a wooden frame, and a minimum of padding. This chair became the oasis in my desert of despair. For some weeks I even sat in it to eat my meals, using a little over-the-lap tray, and resting my arms on the chair arms to take the strain off my back. Only a fellow back patient will realize how painful even raising fork to lips can be unless the elbow is supported in some way. So if you don't have such a comfortable chair, I strongly advise that you acquire one. You deserve it!

Since I was still working at an office job when my back began to act up, I also bought a secretary's chair for use at work. It is a swivel model, adjustable as to height and angle of back. During the several months I was off work, I used my secretary's chair in the dining room. It was surprising the difference it made to swivel the chair instead of my back when getting up and down from the table. You may not want to buy this specialized model in addition to a rocker, but if you happen to have one in your den, give it a try at the dinner table.

You should also pay some attention to the type of lawn chair you have, as getting out into the fresh air and sunshine is important. I found I needed a lawn chair which was more upright and of sturdier construction than the aluminum, frame-webbing type. It goes without saying that chairs built low to the ground are inappropriate for back pain sufferers.

Another useful aid to sitting comfortably is a low footstool. Having the feet slightly raised presses the back more firmly against the chairback for support and raises the knees above hip level which relieves back strain. I have a little stool by my rocker, and another under my typing desk. One woman I know has a portable folding footstool which fits easily into a purse and opens to dimensions of eight inches (20 cm) long, four inches (10 cm) wide and four and one-half inches (11.5 cm) high. It has a leather-like vinyl finish and is very lightweight. She finds it invaluable when travelling by plane, train or bus, or for any activity outside the home which involves sitting for long periods.

Unfortunately, having a proper chair or chairs for use at home doesn't solve the problem of sitting comfortably when you go visiting. For this purpose I acquired a gadget called an "Obus Forme." It is a molded plastic back support, slightly padded, with a washable cover. It is lightweight and portable, and converts an ordinary easy chair into a comfortable seat for the back patient. The Obus Forme is also useful in cars with bucket seats or in any chair which is too deep from front to back. The Obus Forme was invented by a Canadian doctor and is probably available in medical supply centres across Canada. I am not sure whether the distributors have penetrated the American market.

A slightly less effective, but nonetheless helpful, substitute for the Obus Forme is a square foam cushion about two inches (5 cm) thick. I have such a cushion, and for over a year it went with me to theatres, concerts, friends' homes, and doctors' offices, where the chairs are often too deep for comfort. When I don't need the cushion behind my back, I can sit on it to raise me up to almost the height of a normal person!

Another helpful item I recently discovered in a local Back and Body Care shop is an inflatable neck pillow, called "Snooze Eaze," rather like a square collar, which would be especially useful for travelling. You can also get ordinary inflatable pillows which are less bulky than the foam cushion to take on public transit.

As for car seats, the sloped, bucket variety common to most compact cars are very uncomfortable for people with back problems. We had a car with such seats when my trouble began, but later replaced it with one that features bench seats. These are much more supportive and obviate the need for any auxiliary aids. I'm not suggesting that you rush out and buy a new car. But if you are in the market for a vehicle, consider the angle and support factor of the seats.

SAFETY MEASURES

It goes without saying that an osteoporotic must be extremely careful about tripping or falling. Make sure there are no hazards in your home such as loose throw rugs, stairs without hand rails, loose treads, etc. Forget about waxing the floors. Take special precautions in the bathroom. The tub should be equipped either with non-skid decals or a rubber mat with suction cups. I even take my rubber bath mat along when I travel. You may also deem it necessary to have rails installed for support when getting in and out of the bath. These are particularly important for the elderly and for people who live alone.

I've already mentioned the walking cane which is a must in the early stages of disability. And, if you live in a cold climate, you'll need that trusty cane whenever you venture out in the ice and snow. Be sure your winter boots have a deeply grooved, non-slip tread as well.

Another safety consideration is the way you move to perform various tasks. Most back pain sufferers will be familiar with the universal caution to bend the knees when lifting, thus putting the strain on the leg muscles rather than on the spine. But osteoporotics, who aren't likely to be lifting heavy objects, may feel this advice doesn't apply to them. Not so. The bent-knee stance should be adopted even when retrieving an object as light as a feather from the floor or ground. I've forgotten this rule on occasion and have bent instead of squatting to get something from a bottom cupboard. Inevitably a twinge of back pain reminds me of my folly.

Coughing and sneezing can also cause agony to the back patient. If you have enough warning, get on your back with knees bent. If this isn't practical, bend your knees and go into the pelvic tilt (see Chapter 6). To paraphrase a little ditty from a book by Hamilton Hall, orthopedic specialist, "If you can't avoid a cough or sneeze, do the pelvic tilt and bend your knees." It's corny, but if it helps you remember this sage advice, so much the better.

PERSONAL APPEARANCE

A major recovery factor for osteoporotics is combatting the negative psychological aspects of the condition. If you have been blessed with a slim, straight figure all your life, and suddenly your mirror reflects a stooped "little old lady" with a protruding abdomen, it is indeed difficult to muster a positive attitude. But don't despair. There are things you can do, and the sooner you move towards creating a more pleasing self-image, the better. I found a number of measures helpful in counteracting the devastating effects of a radically altered skeletal structure.

The first problem you'll have to deal with is your hair-do. During the acute phase of disability, when raising the arms above shoulder height is sheer torture, grooming your hair can be extremely difficult. I opted for a short, easy-to-manage cut, and was fortunate to find a hairdresser who would come to my home whenever a trim was in order. If your condition makes going to a beauty parlour and performing spinal contortions over the sink next to impossible, seek out a stylist who will make house calls.

Now, about the wardrobe. If your spine has been badly damaged, you'll probably need a proper back support garment. As noted in Chapter I, mine is a sturdily constructed girdle with contoured steel slats running down either side of the spine. It has four straps which tighten over the abdomen, their excess length flopping around in a most annoying way. I solved this problem by sewing a velcro tab to the end of each strap, and its opposite number to the appropriate spot on the girdle. Now I can pull the straps tight and attach the ends firmly. My girdle is a Camp International Ltd. Lumbosacral Support, and it came from a medical supply firm. There are no doubt other equally effective support garments on the market, but I have been more than satisfied with mine. It stood up to over two years of constant wear. I'm now on my second such girdle which, after four years, is still in good shape, as I no longer have to wear it every waking hour.

A few words about laundering your support girdle. Hand washing might promote longer wear, but I found what I think is an easy alternative. Before putting my girdle in the washing machine, I fasten the velcro tabs and enclose the garment in a pillow case secured at the top with a plastic bag fastener. I dry it on a low setting, and it seems to suffer no ill effects. And, if you wear a cotton undershirt under your girdle, it will require less frequent laundering.

I realize that some doctors are against continued use of a support garment, fearing it will make for slack abdominal and back muscles. But I feel that the added activity the support permits, together with faithful adherence to a daily exercise routine, will prevent this from happening. In any case, I find that if I go without my girdle for long periods, my back aches intolerably and I am unable to perform such rigorous chores as scrubbing, vacuuming, or gardening. Whether or not you need such a support garment depends on your degree of disability, and is a matter that should be discussed with your doctor.

Now, a word about the more visible items of clothing. If you've lost a few inches in height and added a comparable number to your waistline, you'll be chagrined to find that few of your clothes fit. But don't despair. You won't have to discard everything. Skirts, for example, may well be salvaged. I found that if I cut three or four inches (7 to 10 cm) off the top and ran an elastic through the new waistband, they looked quite presentable worn with an overblouse or sweater. Tuck-in blouses are a no-no when you no longer have a waistline!

Dresses that are loose fitting can simply be shortened, of course, as can elastic-waisted slacks and skirts. However, you'll likely have to discard slacks with fitted waistbands, and any other items in your wardrobe that hug the figure.

I find shopping for clothes an arduous task at the best of times, and looking for items to suit my altered figure became a formidable challenge. However, I eventually found a few A-line dresses and some with high, low or no waistlines, which are reasonably presentable. Back yokes are excellent if you have a curvature of the upper spine, as they tend to disguise this deformity somewhat.

Now, a word about shoes. It goes without saying that a woman who suffers from osteoporosis doesn't want to go tottering around on spike heels. For walking you'll need the solid support of a sturdy oxford with rubber soles and heels. Well-fitted tennis shoes with molded arches are also good and go well with slacks or shorts. Mine have deeply grooved soles, and I prefer them to the heavier hiking boot for long rambles.

Finding a walking shoe will be easy enough; finding footwear for dressy occasions may be more difficult. Current fashion dictates that dress shoes sport heels guaranteed to throw even a normal spine out of alignment! However, a diligent search should turn up something with a low vamp and a moderate heel to complement a suit or dressy outfit.

Once you've adjusted your wardrobe, along with your sitting, standing, lying, and moving habits, you'll likely find that being osteoporotic isn't the end of the world. By taking care of your external image as best you can, you'll have won half the battle.

But there is still the inner self to deal with. Since you'll probably have to give up the more rigorous activities of your former life, it's essential to find useful occupations and/or hobbies that are compatible with your degree of disability. It's hard to feel good about yourself if you spend your days moping about the house.

When I returned to work, even for a few hours each week, the mental uplift more than compensated for the aching back. And writing this book has added another dimension to my life.

You may not be lucky enough to have a part-time job to return to, but everyone has talent of some kind, and now is a good time to develop yours, be it knitting, sewing, arts and crafts, or whatever. I'd also advise you, as soon as you're up to it, to find some activity, such as volunteer work, which takes you out of the house regularly each week.

I'm not suggesting that you take on a big load all at once. It took me over a year after I became mobile again to work up to my present level of activity. I began slowly, resuming household duties a few at a time, interspersed with periods of rest or sedentary occupations such as knitting or crocheting. The first social venture I undertook was a game of bridge with good friends who would understand if I caved in after a couple of rubbers.

Pacing yourself is the key. Even now I need to lie down for at least an hour sometime during the day. Even short rest periods (10 or 15 minutes) help to relieve back strain after an arduous task. And by resting, I mean lying down with a bolster under the knees and relaxing completely.

Such rests more than pay for themselves in terms of renewed strength and energy. On the whole, I accomplish as much now as I did before my troubles began. I'm reminded of the fable of the hare and the tortoise. I used to tear madly ahead at whatever job I was doing, and often wore myself out in the process. Now I work more calmly, take frequent rests, and try not to get rattled. So remember the old adage, "slow and steady wins the race." It's applicable to anyone recovering from the disabilities associated with osteoporosis.

Chapter 5
Nutrition and Osteoporosis

Nutrition is a large and complex field. The experts have differing opinions, and dietary fads are rampant. The predominant "thin is beautiful" trend has led many girls and young women to diet patterns that may culminate in anorexia, and may set them up for osteoporosis in their middle years. And I am always amazed to hear of an otherwise intelligent person adopting a near-starvation diet without adequate medical supervision.

This chapter does not pretend to present an in-depth study of general nutrition. It will deal mainly with the calcium requirement, since this is the chief concern in the prevention and treatment of osteoporosis.

THE CALCIUM CONNECTION

Ninety-nine per cent of the calcium in your body is stored in the bones and teeth. The other 1 per cent circulates in the blood to regulate such functions as heart rhythm, nerve transmission, and blood clotting. As stated earlier, when the body fails to get enough calcium to fulfil these vital functions, the necessary amount will be released from the bones.

In order to minimize the danger of osteoporosis it is important to maintain an adequate calcium intake *throughout life*. This is important since a prime factor in preventing osteoporosis is achieving peak bone mass by approximately age 35, after which there is a progressive bone loss in both sexes. If you have built up a strong reserve in your "bone bank" you will be better able to withstand the ravages of time.

A nutritious diet throughout life is a prime line of defence against the bone robber. If you are a parent, you have probably urged your children to "drink your milk so you'll have strong bones and teeth." Most parents are very conscientious about their children's diets. Unfortunately, consumption of calcium-rich foods often drops off drastically after adolescence.

Recently my husband had his grade nine science students (aged 13 to 15) keep track of their complete nutrient intake during a typical day. The figures on calcium consumption were startling. Fifty per cent of the girls were getting less than the 1200 mg RDA (recommended daily allowance) as advised by Health and Welfare Canada Dietary Standards for their age and sex. Twenty-five per cent could be classified as very low (under 500 mg, one as low as 74 mg). The boys fared no better, 67 per cent falling below the RDA and 50 per cent receiving half or less of the required amount.

While this was a very small sample, it does serve to illustrate what may well be a common problem in the United States and Canada, and it correlates fairly well with figures shown in Table 1. It would seem that the situation hasn't improved since 1973 when the Nutrition Canada survey was taken.

Table 1
Inadequate Calcium Intake

Age Group and Sex	Percentage in each group deficient in calcium intake
0-4 years	26
5-9 years	44
10-19 years (girls)	62
10-19 years (boys)	51
20-39 years (women)	42
20-39 years (men)	22
40-64 years (women)	44
40-64 years (men)	23
65+ (women)	48
65+ (men)	32
Pregnancy	39

Source: Nutrition Canada, National Survey: Information Canada, Ottawa, 1973.

More recent evidence corroborates these findings. An article in *The Saturday Evening Post* (April 1987) reports on a study done by Dr. John Anderson, Professor of Nutrition at the University of North Carolina. A specialist for 25 years in calcium research, Dr. Anderson investigated the dietary history of his subjects (college women between the ages of 18 and 25) back to their seventh-grade year. He measured their bone mineral content, using a single-photon densitometer, and found that even at such a young age there was noticeably poor mineral content and bone density in the subjects who had a low calcium intake.

The same article reports on another survey done from 1976 to 1980 by the National Center for Health Statistics, which examined the nutritional habits of more than 10,000 Americans selected at random throughout the country. One of the most striking findings of this survey was, again, the low calcium ratings of teen-age girls. Girls aged 12 to 17 averaged only 692 mg of calcium intake a day against the RDA of 1200 mg for their age group.

And Dr. V. Matkovic, of the Department of Rehabilitation Medicine at the University of Washington School of Medicine, Seattle, states that "calcium consumption is probably more important during the period of rapid bone growth—ages 10 to 20—than at any other time in life. During this period, high calcium intake can contribute to osteoporosis prevention."

There is a growing feeling among researchers that the RDA of calcium in both Canada and the United States is too low, particularly for post-menopausal women. Table 2 represents the thinking of some experts in the field.

Another interesting aspect of "the calcium connection" is recent research pointing to a key role for dietary calcium in regulating blood pressure. Findings from a number of studies suggest that low calcium intake can have a deleterious effect, while increasing dietary calcium may protect against hypertension. And, according to Dr. David A. McCarron, Oregon Health Sciences, University of Portland, osteoporotic women have a two- to three-fold increase in incidence of hypertension.

There appear to be conflicting opinions in the literature and among the general public regarding the effect of ingesting too much calcium. Dr. Takuo Fujita examines this factor in great detail in his book *Calcium and Your Health* (pp. 16-17), Japan

Table 2
Recommended Daily Calcium Intake

Age	Calcium per day (mg)
Children:*	
Birth – 0.5 years	360
0.5–1	540
1–10	800
10–18	1,200
Adults** (except pregnant or nursing women):	
Premenopausal women	1,000
Estrogen-treated women	1,000
Postmenopausal women	1,500
Men	1,000

* Based on the most recently available RDAs (1980) developed by the National Academy of Sciences, National Research Council.
** Based on the 1984 NIH Consensus Development Conference Statement on Osteoporosis.

Publications, 1987. Dr. Fujita explains the different effect on the body of calcium ingested orally, and calcium released from the bone.

He points out that dietary calcium deficiency must not be made up simply by drawing calcium from the bone. Besides the deleterious effect on bone mass, such a scenario could have other dangerous aspects. It is imperative that the blood calcium level be kept constant, and any malfunction of the delicate mechanism governing bone resorption could result in a discharge of too much calcium into the bloodstream. Some of this excess may enter the soft tissues, blood vessels, and brain—a frightening proposition, Dr. Fujita states.

He goes on to explain that dietary calcium differs from calcium withdrawn from bone in that normally only the required amount of calcium taken by mouth is absorbed through the intestine. He contends that only if the mechanism controlling calcium absorption by the gut breaks down, is there danger of excessive calcium excretion through the kidneys. If this happens, it could lead to formation of kidney stones. Dr. Fujita concludes, "Normally, however, in most people, intestinal calcium absorption is controlled according to intake . . . and only a small, necessary amount is absorbed from the gut.''

Having, I believe, conclusively proven the case for calcium, let's look at dietary sources of this essential element.

Table 3
Calcium and Protein Content of Some Common Foods

	Amount	Calcium (mg)	Protein (g)
BEVERAGES			
Cocoa made with whole milk	1 cup (250 ml)	314	10
Table wine	²/₅ cup (105 ml)	9	–
Beer	1 bottle	18	1
BREADS AND CEREALS			
Breadcrumbs, grated	1 cup (250 ml)	129	13
Bread, white, enriched	1 slice	20	2
Bread, whole wheat	1 slice	50	3
Granola	¹/₂ cup (125 ml)	34	6
Oats, puffed	1 cup (250 ml)	44	3
Pancakes, buckwheat mix with egg and whole milk	1 oz. (27 g)	59	2
Oatmeal, dry, regular or quick cooking	¹/₂ cup (125 ml)	22	6
COMBINATION DISHES			
Cabbage rolls with meat	approx. 7 oz. (206 g)	66	9
Chili con carne, canned	1 cup (250 ml)	102	28
Lasagna	3¹/₅ oz. (90 g)	108	10
Macaroni and cheese	1 cup (250 ml)	416	19
Spaghetti with meatballs and tomato sauce	1 cup (250 ml)	130	20
Cream of mushroom soup with whole milk	1 cup (250 ml)	201	7

Table 3—Continued

	Amount	Calcium (mg)	Protein (g)
DAIRY PRODUCTS			
Cheese, cheddar, grated	1 tbsp. (15 ml)	50	2
Cheese, cheddar	1½ oz. (45 g)	324	11
Cheese, processed	1½ oz. (45 g)	277	10
Cheese, cottage, 2%	1 cup (250 ml)	161	33
Milk, whole	1 cup (250 ml)	306	8
Milk, 2%	1 cup (250 ml)	315	9
Milk, skim	1 cup (250 ml)	317	9
Milk, dry, skim, reconstituted	1 cup (250 ml)	308	9
Milk, evaporated, 2% fat	1 cup (250 ml)	761	18
Milk, evaporated, 2% fat	1 tbsp. (15 ml)	45	1
Table cream	1 tbsp. (15 ml)	14	tr.
Yogurt, low fat, plain	4⅙ oz. (125 g)	203	6
Yogurt, fruit flavoured	4⅙ oz. (125 g)	176	6
FATS AND OILS			
Butter	1 cup (250 ml)	57	2
Butter	1 tsp. (5 ml)	1	tr.
Margarine, regular	1 cup (250 ml)	48	1
Margarine, regular (no fatty acids)	1 tbsp. (15 ml)	3	tr.
FISH			
Cod, broiled	3 oz. (90 g)	28	26
Sardines, canned	7 medium	393	22
Trout, baked or broiled	3 oz. (90 g)	45	21
Tuna, canned	½ cup (125 ml)	7	26
Salmon, canned with bones	3 oz. (90 g)	100	20
FRUITS			
Apricots, dried	1 cup (250 ml)	105	8
Apricots, cooked	1 cup (250 ml)	67	5
Dates, pitted	1 cup (250 ml)	111	4

Table 3—Continued

	Amount	Calcium (mg)	Protein (g)
Orange	1 medium-sized	54	1
Peaches, dried	1 cup (250 ml)	81	5
Rhubarb, cooked, with sugar	1 cup (250 ml)	224	1
VEGETABLES, COOKED			
Lima beans	1 cup (250 ml)	84	14
Beans, green	1 cup (250 ml)	67	2
Beet greens	1 cup (250 ml)	152	3
Broccoli	1 medium stalk	158	6
Cabbage	1 cup (250 ml)	68	2
Carrots	1 cup (250 ml)	51	1
Onions	1 cup (250 ml)	53	3
Pumpkin, canned	1 cup (250 ml)	60	2
Spinach	1 cup (250 ml)	176	5
Squash, winter, mashed	1 cup (250 ml)	60	4
Turnips, cubed	1 cup (250 ml)	126	2
Zucchini	1 cup (250 ml)	55	2
VEGETABLES, DRY AND NUTS			
Dry beans, white	1 cup (250 ml)	95	15
Beans, canned with pork and tomato sauce	1 cup (250 ml)	146	17
Soybeans, cooked, drained	1 cup (250 ml)	115	17
Chick peas (garbanzo)	1 cup (250 ml)	95	13
Almonds	½ cup (125 ml)	175	14
Brazil nuts	½ cup (125 ml)	128	10
Peanuts, roasted, salted	½ cup (125 ml)	56	19

Source: "Nutrient Value of Some Common Foods." Health & Welfare Canada, 1979.

Notes: This table constitutes a sketchy guide, confined mostly to foods with a reasonably high calcium content. Protein content is given to illustrate how much of that element is available from non-meat sources, and because of the suspected effect of excess protein on calcium absorption. Recommended daily allowance of protein: 56 g for an adult male, 41 g for an adult female.

Milk and milk products are widely recognized as the chief dietary source of calcium. As you will see from Table 3, four glasses of skim milk would provide the bulk of your daily calcium requirement. But if you balk at the thought of drinking milk at all, let alone four glasses a day, don't despair. There are other routes to follow. Foods equivalent in calcium content to one glass of milk include 1½ oz. (40 g) cheddar cheese, 1 cup (250 ml) yogurt, 2 cups (500 ml) cottage cheese, ½ cup (125 ml) evaporated milk, 2¼ oz. (64 g) sardines, or 4 oz. (113 g) canned salmon (with bones and oil). Still, fluid milk remains the most available source of calcium, and it is also high in other essential nutrients. You should, if at all possible, include milk in your diet. If you are one of those unfortunate people who have a lactose intolerance (lack of the enzyme lactase necessary for the digestion of milk), ask your doctor about a product called LactAid which assists in the digestion of lactose.

You may have heard recent rumours that homogenization and pasteurization destroy the calcium content in milk. Not so. An eminent research nutritionist, who does not wish to be quoted, assured me that loss of calcium caused by these processes would not be greater than 1 or 2 per cent. And a recent publication, *Calcium: A Summary of Current Research for the Health Professional*, states: "According to animal experiments, the heat treatment of pasteurization does not significantly affect the availability of calcium in milk." Nor, the article continues, does homogenization affect the bioavailability of calcium in milk. It concludes: "Pasteurized, homogenized cow's milk is regarded as a significant source of calcium, not only because of its high content of calcium, but also because of the excellent bioavailability of this mineral in milk."

If, however, you cannot include fluid milk in your diet, you can usually add the powdered skim variety to soups, puddings, meatloaves, casseroles, etc. (unless, of course, you are allergic to milk or lactose intolerant). Powdered skim milk contains all the nutrients of whole milk with the exception of fat, and it is, in fact, slightly higher in calcium than whole milk. Skim milk powder has been a staple in our household for many years. Bill and I drink the reconstituted product, which appalls our finicky children. But we find that after a few hours refrigeration, it is quite palatable, and its use is highly economical.

A WORD ABOUT SNACKS

Studying nutrition has turned me into a veritable fanatic about avoiding unhealthy between-meal snacks. We used to put out chips and salted nuts, or other such items, to nibble at the bridge table. Now we serve dried fruit or a mixture of raw almonds and raisins. It's amazing how quickly the palate can adjust to changes in taste sensations. I've reduced the salt and sugar content of cooked and baked items by at least one-half, and have come to much prefer a nutty taste to a sweet one, or a spiced or herb-flavoured dish to a highly salted one.

Adjusting to other healthy snack foods such as raw or canned fruit, yogurt with fruit, raw vegetable sticks with dip, cherry tomatoes, cheese slices alone or on whole grain crackers, is a relatively easy matter. The trick is to have such items available. I dry large amounts of fruit during the summer and fall, so that these tasty morsels are always handy on the shelf. And when preparing vegetables for dinner, I wash and slice a few extra pieces, which are kept in a tightly covered fridge dish. I, for one, would be too lazy to wash and cut a few "veggies" whenever I felt the need of a snack, but if they're already prepared, what could be easier?

For a healthy drink, you might try a "smoothie" made from plain yogurt and any combination of fresh or canned fruit whirled in the blender. This tasty, calcium-laden drink lends itself to all sorts of innovations. Then, there's the old standby, cocoa. If you don't have to count calories, you might make it with evaporated milk which has a very high calcium content.

There are many possibilities for healthy snacks and drinks. Here are a few for the budget-wise.

INSTANT COCOA MIX

¾ cup (190 ml) cocoa
4 cups (1000 ml) instant skim milk powder
½ cup (125 ml) sugar

Mix these ingredients together well (sift cocoa if lumpy) for bulk supply.

To make up one mug of cocoa, combine 3 tbsp. (45 ml) of the mix with 2 tbsp. (30 ml) evaporated milk. Mix well. Add boiling water to fill mug.

HOME-MADE YOGURT

1 package unflavoured gelatin (dissolve in ½ cup [125 ml] boiling water)
2 cups (500 ml) lukewarm water
1 cup (250 ml) instant skim milk powder
3 tbsp. (45 ml) plain yogurt (for starter)

Add powdered milk to lukewarm water. Stir well. Add gelatin mixture and yogurt starter.

I make mine in a quart sealer (1 litre) which I cover and place in the oven with the light on for several hours until it reaches proper consistency (until it has "yoged" as my daughter says!).

The following are a few suggested menus with a reasonable calcium content:

BREAKFAST

Food serving	Calcium content (mg)
(1) 1 medium orange	54
1 cup (250 ml) whole grain porridge	53
with ½ cup (125 ml) milk (whole)	150
1 cup (250 ml) coffee with 2 tbsp.	
(30 ml) evaporated milk	90
	347
(2) 1 glass (250 ml) orange juice	29
1 corn meal muffin, buttered	100
1½ oz. (45 g) cheddar cheese	324
1 cup (250 ml) tea	–
	453
(3) ½ grapefruit	10
1 cup (250 ml) cream of wheat	18
with ½ cup (125 ml) whole milk	150
1 cup (250 ml) coffee with	
2 tbsp. (30 ml) evaporated milk	90
	268

(4) 1 cup (250 ml) grape juice   28
    1 cup (250 ml) puffed wheat   7
       with 1 cup (250 ml) whole milk   300
    1 corn meal muffin, buttered   100
    1 cup (250 ml) tea   –
                                                           ___
                                                           435

(5) 1 glass (250 ml) apple juice   15
    2 slices whole wheat toast   100
    4⅙ oz. (125 g) fruit flavoured
       yogurt   176
    1 cup (250 ml) coffee with
       2 tbsp. (30 ml) evaporated milk   90
                                                           ___
                                                           381

(6) 1 glass (250 ml) orange juice   29
    2 buckwheat pancakes
       (4¼ in. [11 cm] diameter)   118
       with 1 tbsp. (15 ml) butter   3
       3 tbsp. (45 ml) maple syrup   62
    1 cup (250 ml) coffee with
       2 tbsp. (30 ml) evaporated milk   90
                                                           ___
                                                           302

(7) 1 medium orange   54
    1 egg, boiled   28
    1 slice whole wheat toast   50
    1 cup (250 ml) cocoa made with
       whole milk   314
                                                           ___
                                                           446

LUNCH

Food serving	Calcium content (mg)
(1) 1 glass (250 ml) 2% milk	315
5 oz. (125 g) low-fat yogurt	203
2 bran muffins with butter	69
1 banana	10
	597

(2) Toasted cheese sandwich:
   2 slices whole wheat bread   100
   3 oz. (85 g) processed cheese   554
   raw carrot sticks (1 medium carrot)   18
   1 cup (250 ml) tea   –
                                         672

(3) 3 oz. (85 g) canned salmon
   (with bones)   372
   1 slice whole wheat bread   50
   1 small tomato   20
   ¼ cucumber   13
   1 glass (250 ml) 2% milk   315
                                         770

(4) 2 squares, 2 in. (5 cm) cornbread   174
   ½ cup (125 ml) 2% cottage cheese   80
   1 stick raw celery   16
   1 cup (250 ml) Ovaltine made with
     whole milk   333
                                         603

(5) 2 slices rye bread   54
   1 cup (250 ml) chicken soup made
     with whole milk   181
   1 cup (250 ml) fruit cocktail   24
   1 glass (250 ml) 2% milk   315
                                         574

(6) Swiss cheese sandwich:
   2 oz. (56 g) Swiss cheese   540
   2 slices whole wheat bread   100
   tomato and lettuce   20
   1 cup (250 ml) tea   –
                                         660

(7) 1 cup (250 ml) clam chowder   91
     2 slices rye bread   54
     1 medium raw pear   13
     1 glass (250 ml) 2% milk   315
                                 473

DINNER

Food serving	*Calcium content (mg)*
(1) 1 cup (250 ml) spaghetti and meatballs with tomato sauce	130
3 tbsp. (45 ml) grated Parmesan cheese	207
Vegetable salad:	
1 cup (250 ml) spinach	30
½ cup (125 ml) mushrooms	1
½ cup (125 ml) alfalfa sprouts	25
½ cup (125 ml) broccoli	72
¼ cup (62 ml) onion	15
2 oz. (56 g) cubed tofu*	75
1 tbsp. (15 ml) blue cheese dressing	12
1 cup (250 ml) canned apricots	30
1 cup (250 ml) tea	–
	597
(2) ½ baked chicken breast	9
1 cup (250 ml) steamed green beans	62
1 medium baked potato	14
with 2 tbsp. (30 ml) plain yogurt and chives	50
1 cup (250 ml) raw raspberries	29
with ½ cup (125 ml) coffee cream	134
1 glass (250 ml) 2% milk	315
	613

*Tofu is a soy bean product, rich in calcium (2 oz. = 75 mg) and protein. It is tasteless by itself, but tends to absorb the flavour of foods with which it is mixed and makes a nourishing addition to such items as soups, salad dressings, vegetable dips, etc.

(3) Shrimp stir-fry with vegetables:
4 oz. (113 g) fresh shrimp | 72
one 5½ in. (14 cm) stalk broccoli | 103
1 stalk celery | 16
1 cup (250 ml) kale | 206
½ cup (125 ml) green beans | 30
½ cup (125 ml) brown rice | 9
1 tbsp. (15 ml) sesame oil and
soy sauce to taste | –
1 cup (250 ml) canned plums | 23
1 glass (250 ml) 2% milk | 315
774

(4) 4 oz. (113 g) poached salmon | 90
1 cup (250 ml) cooked chard | 106
1 cup (250 ml) cooked carrots | 51
1 medium baked potato | 14
1 tbsp. (15 ml) butter | 3
½ cup (125 ml) baked custard | 147
1 glass (250 ml) 2% milk | 315
726

(5) Stir-fry chicken broccoli:
4 oz. (113 g) cubed chicken | 10
2 stalks, 5½-in. (14 cm) broccoli | 309
2 tbsp (30 ml) sesame oil | –
2 tbsp. (30 ml) soy sauce | 30
½ cup (125 ml) brown rice | 9
1 cup (250 ml) fresh strawberries | 33
with ½ cup (125 ml) coffee cream | 134
1 glass (250 ml) 2% milk | 315
840

(6) 4 oz. (113 g) broiled hamburger | 14
on bun with | 40
1 oz. (28 g) cheese | 195
Salad:
1 cup (250 ml) romaine lettuce | 15
½ cup (125 ml) cabbage | 17
1 tomato | 20

1 tbsp. (15 ml) oil and vinegar	–
1 sliced raw peach with	16
½ cup (125 ml) coffee cream	134
1 glass (250 ml) 2% milk	315
	766

(7) 1 medium baked potato with	9
2 tbsp. (30 ml) plain yogurt and chives	50
½ cup (125 ml) steamed beets	12
1 tbsp. (15 ml) butter	3
1 slice, 2 oz. (56 g) roast beef	5
½ cup (125 ml) orange sherbet	37
1 glass (250 ml) 2% milk	315
	431

DIETARY ANALYSIS

In order to ascertain my calcium and protein intake, I kept strict track of my diet for a week recently. It was surprising to find that, although I'm a moderate meat eater, my protein intake was above the 41g RDA in each of the seven days. My calcium intake, without any special dietary adjustments, averaged about 1000 mg and required only a modest supplement to bring it in line with recommended requirements.

Table 4 shows a sample day's diet, deliberately calculated to pump up the calcium content. It should be noted that the total amounts of both calcium and protein shown in this table are far above the recommended daily requirements. The table is included merely as an example of the quantity of calcium easily obtainable from dietary sources. I included protein content to illustrate how a normal North American diet frequently contains over twice the RDA of this nutrient. This is an atypical day, however, in that it includes such items as white sauce and sardines which would not likely form part of the daily routine. Who wouldn't balk at sardine sandwiches seven days a week? But even if you subtract these two items, you still come up with 1364 mg of calcium. If you further subtract the fluid milk and cocoa, the calcium intake would be reduced to 742 mg. It is evident from this exercise that by including such high calcium foods as sardines and fluid milk, it is easy to reach the RDA of calcium from dietary means alone. Without such items, a supplement would be required.

Table 4
One Day's High-calcium Diet

Breakfast	Calcium (mg)	Protein (g)
1 medium orange	54	1
½ cup (125 ml) oatmeal porridge	22	6
with ½ cup (125 ml) whole milk	153	4
1 slice whole wheat toast	50	3
with 1 tsp. (5 ml) butter	1	tr.
1 cup (250 ml) coffee		
with 2 tbsp. (30 ml)		
evaporated milk	90	2
Mid-morning		
1 glass (250 ml) apple juice	16	tr.
Lunch		
7 medium sardines	393	22
2 slices whole wheat bread	100	6
2 tsp. (10 ml) butter	2	tr.
1 cup (250 ml) powdered skim milk	308	9
6 raw carrot sticks	18	1
Mid-afternoon		
1 medium banana	10	1
clear tea		
Dinner		
1 medium baked potato	9	3
½ cup (125 ml) steamed broccoli	72	2
½ cup (125 ml) white sauce	152	1
½ cup (125 ml) steamed beets	12	1
1 tbsp. (15 ml) butter		
(on vegetables)	3	tr.
1 slice, 2 oz. (56 g) roast beef	5	13
½ cup (125 ml) orange sherbet	37	1

Evening

¼ cup (63 ml) shelled raw almonds	88	7
1 cup (250 ml) cocoa made with whole milk	314	10
Total:	1909	93

CALCIUM SUPPLEMENTS

While most doctors agree that it is better to get your calcium from dietary sources, supplements are valuable when this is not practical. You will find a mind-boggling array of calcium supplements on the shelves of any pharmacy, all available without a prescription. It is not wise, however, to take calcium without a doctor's advice. Expert opinion varies on the danger of too much calcium. Some believe that as much as 2500 mg a day produces no ill effects, while others are cautious of amounts in excess of 1500 mg a day. Dr. Recker, of Creighton University, states that excess amounts of calcium can reduce bone remodelling, and he suggests that consumption in excess of 1500 mg a day be avoided.

There are a few basic facts you should be aware of when shopping for a calcium supplement. Most contain one of three calcium compounds—calcium lactate, calcium gluconate, or calcium carbonate. These compounds vary widely in the amount of elemental calcium they contain. Elemental calcium is the amount of the nutrient the body actually absorbs, and it is elemental calcium you must use in calculating your daily intake. The percentage of elemental calcium contained in each of the three compounds is as follows: calcium carbonate—40%; calcium lactate—13%; calcium gluconate—9%. This means that if, for example, your doctor prescribed a 500 mg a day supplement, you would have to take considerably larger quantities of calcium gluconate or calcium lactate than of calcium carbonate in order to obtain the 500 mg of elemental calcium. You might mention this factor when discussing calcium supplements with your physician. He or she will be able to explain to you the antacid quality of calcium carbonate which may have a bearing on its suitability in your case.

Calcium supplements also come in a variety of forms. You can get them in liquid form, as chewable tablets, or as effervescent tablets which dissolve easily in water or fruit juice. There are also "chelated" calcium tablets. Chelation anchors the calcium to other chemicals which is supposed to improve absorption. *Consumer Reports* (October 1984) advises, however, that according to their medical consultants, "chelation does nothing more than jack up the price of the tablets."

Then there are calcium supplements which may be contaminated with lead and should definitely be avoided. These are manufactured from crushed cattle bones (bone meal) or from a form of limestone (dolomite). The United States Food and Drug Administration has warned doctors and the general public about these products. *Consumer Reports* (September 1982) offers a comprehensive report on lead-contaminated calcium supplements.

The October 1984 *Consumer Reports* article cited earlier contains a table on calcium supplements which gives the price per 1000 mg of elemental calcium for each brand. These, of course, are United States products and prices. With the idea of compiling a similar table for Canadian products, I descended on a local pharmacy armed with notebook and pen. Some two months later, when replenishing my own calcium supplement, I found that all the prices had risen, rendering those in my carefully constructed table obsolete. I decided, therefore, to omit the price column. The table will still be helpful in that it shows, at a glance, the elemental calcium content per tablet or teaspoon of various brands.

Table 5
Some Calcium Supplements Available in Canada

Brand	Calcium form	Elemental calcium content (mg per tablet or liquid equivalent)
*Tums, unflavoured	Ca. carbonate	200 per tablet
*Tums, extra strength	Ca. carbonate	300 per tablet
Oscal 500	Ca. carbonate	500 per tablet
*Biocal	Ca. carbonate	500 per tablet
Natural Source Calcium 250	Ca. carbonate	250 per tablet

*Calcium Sandoz		
Gramcal	⎧(Ca. carbonate ⎨(Ca. gluconate ⎩(Ca. lactate	1000 per tablet
Calcium Sandoz		
Forte	⎧(Ca. carbonate ⎨(Ca. gluconate ⎩(Ca. lactate	500 per tablet
*Sandoz Syrup	⎰(Ca. gluconate ⎱(Ca. lactate	110 per tsp. (5 ml)
Calcium Stanley	⎰(Ca. gluconate ⎱(Ca. glucoheptonate	100 per tsp. (5 ml)
Wampoles Calcium Gluconate	Ca. gluconate	60 per tablet
Adams Calcium Gluconate	Ca. gluconate	60 per tablet
Adams Calcium Lactate	Ca. lactate	84 per tablet
Life Calcium Lactate	Ca. lactate	84 per tablet
Life Liquid Calcium	Not given	100 per tsp. (5 ml)
Caltrate (Lederle)	Ca. carbonate	600 per tablet

*Labelled low sodium content.

Some Calcium Supplements Available in the United States

Brand	Calcium form	Elemental calcium content (mg per tablet)
Tums antacid (Morcliffe-Thayer)	Ca. carbonate	200
Caltrate (Lederle)	Ca. carbonate	600
Calcium carbonate (Lilly)	Ca. carbonate	260
Biocal (Miles)	Ca. carbonate	500
Alka-2 antacid (Miles)	Ca. carbonate	200
Os-Cal (Marion)	Ca. carbonate	500

Calcium lactate (Gen. Nutrition Corp.)	Ca. lactate	100
Natural calcium lactate (Schiff)	Ca. lactate	100
Formula 31 (Plus)	Ca. lactate	83
Calcium lactate (Lilly)	Ca. lactate	84
Calcium gluconate (Pioneer)	Ca. gluconate	62
Calcium gluconate (Lilly)	Ca. gluconate	47

Source: *Consumer Reports*, October 1984, Vol. 49, No. 10

Of course, this table does not cover every form and brand of calcium supplement on the market. You and your doctor should consider all products readily available before reaching a decision as to which is best for you.

In order to arrive at the correct dosage of calcium supplement required (if any) a full dietary analysis is recommended. I did such an analysis for myself, using tables provided in the Health and Welfare Canada publication, "Nutrient Value of Some Common Foods." You might find it easier to consult a registered dietician.

There are conflicting opinions as to the best time of day to take your calcium supplement. My most recent source recommends mealtimes or up to one and a half hours after meals. Taking the supplement with a glass of water aids the absorption process.

FACTORS AFFECTING CALCIUM ABSORPTION

PROTEIN

You will note that I included protein content in Tables 3 and 4. This is included because excess protein is believed to have an adverse effect on calcium absorption. Opinions among clinicians vary as to how much excess protein is required to produce this effect. But it is quite clear that North Americans as a whole consume considerably more than the RDA of 41 g a day for an adult female, 56 g a day for an adult male.

ALUMINUM

In Chapter 2 we mentioned that the aluminum contained in certain antacids had a deleterious effect on calcium absorption. A report by Dr. Herta Spencer, Lois Kramer, and Dace Osis examines, in great detail, studies carried out in this field. In connection with one such project they report: ". . . other investigators have shown that phosphorus depletion, induced by large doses of aluminum-containing antacids is associated with an increase in urinary calcium. The present study has shown that even small doses of these antacids have a similar effect."

Then there is the startling case of a 60-year-old woman admitted to Strong Memorial Hospital, Rochester, N.Y., complaining of great pain in her legs and scarcely able to walk. She was diagnosed as osteoporotic and it was discovered that for 12 years she had been taking an antacid containing aluminum. Urine analysis showed an extremely high rate of calcium excretion and no phosphate. The antacid was discontinued, and after one month she began to notice dramatic improvement.

Some widely used antacids containing aluminum are: Amphojel, Delcid, Di-Gel, Gaviscon, Gelusil, Maalox, Mylanta, Riopan, Rolaids, Simeco. Antacids without aluminum include: Alka-Seltzer, Alka-2, Bisodol, Citrocarbonate, Eno, Marblen, Percy Medicine, Titralac, Tums (*Stand Tall! Every Woman's Guide to Preventing Osteoporosis*, pp. 107-108).

Sometimes labels on pharmaceutical products are difficult to read, because of the small print, and difficult for the layperson to interpret. If you are in doubt about the ingredients in an antacid, ask your doctor or pharmacist.

VITAMIN D

As previously stated, adequate vitamin D is required to aid calcium absorption. *Nutrition Quarterly* (Vol. 7, No. 4, 1983), gives a detailed analysis of vitamin D requirements. It quotes the Canadian RDA as 100 IU and the United States RDA as 400 IU. It appears that the experts disagree on the optimum daily requirement. Some feel that for older people, the RDA should be increased to 600-800 IU. Clinicians do agree, however, that excessive amounts of vitamin D may be associated with increased bone resorption. The American Society for Bone and Mineral Research recommends avoidance of amounts in excess of 1000 IU a day.

Suppose your doctor decides that you should take the middle way, and consume 400-600 IU a day of vitamin D. What are the sources of this vitamin? Most of us can remember the traumatic childhood experience of gagging on a daily spoonful of cod liver oil. Fortunately, you won't have to resort to such distasteful measures. While natural dietary sources of vitamin D are limited, all milk sold in North America, including the powdered variety, is fortified with 400 IU of vitamin D per quart (litre). So you get approximately 100 IU of vitamin D in every glass (250 ml) of milk. Sunshine is also an excellent source of vitamin D, but it is difficult to estimate the amount you're getting from this source. Many multi-vitamins include 400 IU of vitamin D per tablet. But here again, do not dose yourself without the advice of a physician.

VITAMIN A

Vitamin A is needed for normal bone growth. The article in *Nutrition Quarterly* referred to above mentions that excess amounts of vitamin A can stimulate bone resorption. According to the American Society for Bone and Mineral Research, more than 5000 IU a day may stimulate bone loss. Their recommended daily allowance is 4000 IU. Again, self-medication with vitamin A should be avoided.

VITAMIN C

This vitamin is needed to form the protein network in bones. I found only two references in my sources to vitamin C as it relates to bone. *Postgraduate Medicine* (Vol. 63, No. 3, March 1978) states: ". . . adequate intake of vitamin C is essential for biosynthesis of collagen" (the manufacturing of collagen, a protein which is an important constituent of bone). Health expert and author Jane E. Brody comments: "consumption of foods rich in vitamin C . . . along with calcium-containing foods may increase your body's ability to absorb calcium." Health and Welfare Canada's RDA for vitamin C is 30 mg.

SODIUM

It is widely accepted that too much salt can affect blood pressure, increasing the risk of heart and vascular disease. The role this element plays in osteoporosis is less publicized. Nevertheless, there is evidence that calcium excretion in the urine is directly related to the quantity of sodium in the diet because you excrete calcium along with the excess sodium.

The Food and Nutrition Board of the National Academy of Sciences (U.S.) recommends a daily intake of 1100-3300 mg of sodium. The American Heart Association says the maximum should be 2000 mg a day. According to a publication of the National Dairy Council, however, Americans consume an average of 3600-5850 mg a day. Another source makes the even more startling statement that most of us consume ten to twenty times as much sodium as we need (*Stand Tall! Every Woman's Guide to Preventing Osteoporosis*, p. 100).

Whatever the estimates, it is widely accepted that North Americans as a whole consume far too much salt. A cursory glance at Table 6 will show you why.

Table 6
Sodium Content of Some Common Foods

	Sodium content (mg)
Milk group	
1 cup (250 ml) skim milk	126
1 cup (250 ml) yogurt	159
1 oz. (28 g) cheddar cheese	176
Meat group	
1 egg	69
3 oz. (84 g) chicken	69
3 oz. (84 g) beef	55
2 slices bacon	274
1 frankfurter	639
3 oz. (84 g) tuna	303
3 oz. (84 g) canned ham	1114
Grain group	
1 slice whole wheat bread	132
¾ cup (188 ml) oatmeal	1
¾ cup (188 ml) cream of wheat	126
1 cup (250 ml) cornflakes	256
1 waffle	275

Combination dishes

Fast food hamburger, regular	461
jumbo	990
Home-baked pot pie, 8 oz. (225 g)	644
Home-made chow mein, 1 cup (250 ml)	718
Canned spaghetti and meatballs, 1 cup (250 ml)	942
Pizza with sausage, 2 slices, 7 oz. (200 g)	967
Canned chicken noodle soup, 1 cup (250 ml)	1107

Spreads and condiments

Butter, 1 tsp. (5 ml)	41
Margarine, 1 tsp. (5 ml)	47
Prepared mustard, 1 tsp. (5 ml)	65
Mayonnaise, 1 tbsp. (15 ml)	78
Italian dressing, 1 tbsp. (15 ml)	116
French dressing, 1 tbsp. (15 ml)	214
Catsup, 1 tbsp. (15 ml)	156
Tartar sauce, 1 tbsp. (15 ml)	182
Monosodium glutamate (MSG), 1 tsp. (5 ml)	492
Soy sauce, 1 tbsp. (15 ml)	1029
Bouillon, 1 cube	1152
Table salt, 1 tsp. (5 ml)	1938

You will note that one teaspoon of salt contains nearly 2000 mg of sodium. So you could easily throw away your salt shaker and still get more than the required RDA. If you are concerned about osteoporosis, it would be wise to avoid foods which are high in salt and low in calcium. Instant meals and processed foods should also be kept to a minimum. When you cook for yourself, you have control over the amount of salt. You need not become an anti-salt fanatic. But be aware of the sodium factor and of a few simple tricks for cutting down on your use of this element. For instance, it's a relatively simple matter to cut by half or even by three-quarters the amount of salt called for in any recipe. I've been doing this for years and my family hasn't even noticed the difference. As stated earlier, I tend to use more spices and herbs and less salt in main course dishes. And I'm still working on educating Bill not to buy those salt-laden munchies he's so fond of!

OXALATES, PHYTATES, AND FIBRE

Oxalates are compounds which abound in green vegetables. Phytates, phosphorus-containing compounds, are found mostly in the outer husks of cereal grains. Both oxalates and phytates, along with fibre, decrease the absorption of calcium to some extent. You should not, however, avoid high fibre foods; they are necessary for normal intestinal function and for the other nutrients they contain. And, most likely, you are getting too little rather than too much fibre. Just don't count too heavily on green vegetables and whole grains when calculating your calcium intake. Dairy products remain the most reliable and easily absorbed dietary source of calcium. Remember that in order to fully utilize your calcium, whether from dietary sources or from a supplement, it is best to avoid combining it with high fibre foods at the same meal.

PHOSPHATES

I found considerable differences of opinion among my sources as to the effect of the phosphates and the calcium-phosphate ratio on bone. For example, Dr. Notelovitz, co-author of *Stand Tall! Every Woman's Guide to Preventing Osteoporosis* (pp. 105-106), while admitting that there is uncertainty as to the role of the calcium-phosphate ratio, advises consuming at least as much calcium as phosphorus. He gives a comprehensive table showing the ratio of these two elements in various foods. But almost every item listed contains more phosphorus than calcium. The few exceptions are canned green beans, cheddar cheese, soft ice cream, lettuce, and spinach. It would appear, therefore, that you would have to consume an extremely monotonous diet and one lacking many essential nutrients, if you wished to keep your calcium-phosphate ratio in balance. The table is useful, however, in that it points out the items with extremely high phosphorus content. All meats fall into this category, and they have the added disadvantage of being low in calcium. Unfortunately, most of the high-calcium foods such as dairy products and certain fish, are also

91

high in phosphate. One can see from this brief outline, that the whole area of calcium-phosphorus ratio is fraught with difficulty.

No need to despair, however. Studies by other researchers discredit the idea that phosphates have a negative bearing on calcium excretion, calcium absorption, or bone mass. Dr. Spencer, Lois Kramer, and Dace Osis have reported extensively on such studies. They cite one finding that phosphate supplements tended to promote fracture healing and to decrease urinary calcium excretion, and that phosphate intake of up to 2000 mg a day did not interfere with intestinal absorption of calcium. They conclude: ". . . in view of the fact that the high phosphorus intake in man and widely varying ca-ph [calcium-phosphate] ratios did not interfere with intestinal absorption of calcium, it appears that the dietary ca-ph [calcium-phosphate] ratio in humans does not play an important role in terms of utilization and retention of calcium." They go on to cite three separate studies suggesting that added phosphate may decrease urinary calcium excretion as a consequence of increased bone formation and bone mineralization.

It would appear that the daily calcium-phosphate ratio is another of those grey areas where it would be wise to steer a middle course.

So it is with the whole field of nutrition. We are inundated with conflicting advice—vegetarians advocating their lifestyle, health food stores promoting their products, one dietary fad replacing another in rapid succession. No wonder the layperson trying to decide on a healthy diet may throw up his/her hands in despair.

My own belief is that if you pay attention to including foods from each of the four groups (dairy products, bread and cereals, fruits and vegetables, meat and alternatives) in your daily diet, if you cut down on salt and sugar and conform to the RDA for calcium, you won't go too far wrong. My brother once accused me of being "moderate to the extreme." When it comes to charting a safe dietary course through the shoals and rapids of conflicting advice, I gladly plead guilty to that charge.

Chapter 6
Exercise:
A Key Factor

Throughout the book I have stressed the importance of a regular exercise program. Such a program fulfils a dual function.

1. It is vital for anyone suffering vertebral damage to keep the supporting musculature in top shape to lessen the strain on the spinal column.
2. There is evidence that weight-bearing exercise enhances bone formation and that bones, like muscles, can atrophy if they aren't subjected to stress.

I had intended in this chapter to detail, with diagrams, the quite rigorous exercise regimen I now follow. But the physiotherapist I consulted on this chapter dissuaded me. She felt that some readers might attempt the routines on their own, ignoring the warning to do them only with the approval of a doctor or therapist. Any adoption of an unsanctioned program, she felt, could well lead to spinal damage.

I outline here the "early exercise" program my physiotherapist recommended while I was still in the acute phase of disability, but not the advanced routine.

Bear in mind, however, that osteoporosis affects different people in different ways. It is absolutely essential to seek medical approval before starting even these mild routines. I suggest you go over each exercise with your clinician, and be guided by him/her as to which ones are suitable for you at present, and how soon you should progress to more strenuous routines.

In my own case, I proceeded with extreme caution in building my program to its present level. I did each new exercise only once or twice the first day, and very slowly and carefully at that. I still perform all exercises in bed, on a firm mattress which provides support and cushioning. I like to compare the brittle bones of osteoporotics with fine china. When you pack a barrel of dishes you put a cushioning of excelsior in the bottom to act as a shock absorber. The mattress on which you perform your exercise routine is the shock absorber which prevents spinal damage.

The way you do the exercises is important, too. You must avoid jerky movements, proceeding always with a slow, smooth rhythm and breathing evenly. Often when doing exercises which call for rigorous contraction of abdominal muscles there is a tendency to hold the breath. Don't do it! Except for the deep breathing exercises themselves, you should breathe normally throughout. It is also a good idea to relax completely for a few seconds and take a couple of deep breaths after each routine.

To recapitulate, in order to ensure that your exercise program is safe and helpful for you:

1. Consult your doctor and/or therapist before beginning.
2. Proceed slowly and carefully as, under professional guidance, you add more difficult routines.
3. Always avoid jerky movements.
4. Breathe naturally.
5. Relax between exercises.
6. Adopt a positive attitude. Enjoy your exercise program rather than regarding it as a chore.

KEY TO POSITION TERMINOLOGY

Starting position: Lie on your back on a firm mattress, knees bent, feet flat on the bed, arms at sides. Put a small pillow under your neck for comfort and support. A feather or foam-chip pillow is preferable to the more rigid solid-foam type. (See Figure 5.)

Pelvic tilt position: see Exercise 2.

Modified pelvic tilt: Assume starting position, contract abdominal muscles, press small of back firmly against mattress, but keep buttocks flat on bed.

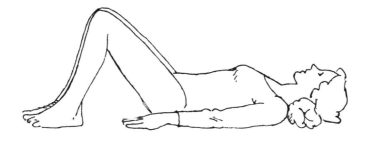

Figure 5. Starting Position for All Exercises

EARLY EXERCISES

These can be started, subject to medical approval, during the acute phase of disability. Unless otherwise stated, start with one or two repeats of each exercise the first day, and gradually work up to ten.

EXERCISE 1: DEEP BREATHING

Assume starting position. You may wish to place a bolster under your knees for more comfort. Breathe deeply, inhaling slowly to the maximum. Hold for three seconds (count "one and two and three and" etc.). Exhale slowly.

EXERCISE 2: PELVIC TILT

(An important routine to master, as many of the following exercises involve this manoeuvre). Assume starting position. Contract abdominal muscles firmly, tighten buttocks, anal and vaginal muscles, flattening the small of the back against the mattress.

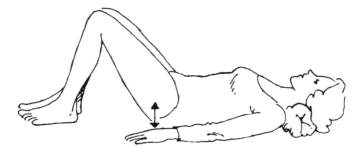

Figure 6. Exercise 2: Pelvic Tilt

Buttocks (but not hips) will be fractionally raised off the mattress. Hold for six seconds. Relax. A version of this exercise can be performed from a sitting or standing position, and it is excellent for relieving back strain.

EXERCISE 3: LEG BENDS

Adopt modified pelvic tilt. Grasp right knee with both hands and slowly bring the knee up until thigh rests on chest (or as close as you can come). Hold for six seconds. Lower right leg to starting position. Repeat exercise with left leg. Work up to ten repeats with each leg.

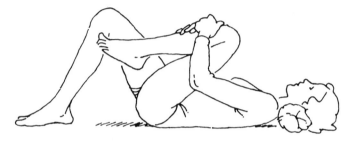

Figure 7. Exercise 3: Leg Bends

EXERCISE 4: KNEE PRESS AGAINST RESISTANCE

Assume modified pelvic tilt. Raise left foot an inch or two off the bed. Place right hand on left knee and push, while resisting with left leg. Hold for six seconds. Repeat with left hand pressing and right leg resisting.

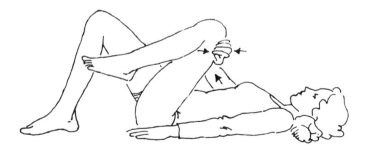

Figure 8. Exercise 4: Knee Press Against Resistance

EXERCISE 5: PARTIAL SIT-UPS

Assume modified pelvic tilt. Slowly extend arms over knees as you raise your head and upper back from the pillow. Hold for three seconds. Extend arms to right of knees. Hold for three seconds. Extend arms to left of knees. Hold for three seconds. Relax. Work up to ten repeats of the entire routine. This exercise may be difficult at first. Don't try for too great an extension to begin with. If you are still experiencing muscle spasm, omit the extensions to right and left.

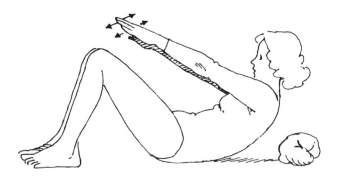

Figure 9. Exercise 5: Partial Sit-ups

EXERCISE 6: DEEP BREATHING WITH OUTWARD EXPANSION

As in Exercise 1, but this time strive to push lungs and chest muscles outwards. At the risk of sounding like a bra commercial, I urge you to lift and separate the breasts!

These six exercises constitute the program I adopted during the acute phase of disability. If you are suffering severe back pain, it is important not to overdo even these mild routines. Better to do them fewer times at each session, but do at least three sessions a day.

At first it may seem that such mild exercise is accomplishing nothing, but rest assured that it is. And remember, the faithful performance of these mild routines will enable you to progress to more difficult manoeuvres as you become stronger. DON'T GIVE UP!

ADVANCED ROUTINE

My current rigorous exercise routine is proof of what patience and persistence can accomplish.

In addition to the six exercises detailed above, I now do arm stretches with and without weights, ankle circling, side knee bends, leg raises (both single and together), forearm pushes, hand cross-overs, weightlifting with legs, knee-chin touches, and head press against resistance, among others. Only a slow and steady build-up over a period of some two years enabled me to progress to this level. Again, such an advanced routine should not be attempted without consulting a doctor. All the more difficult manoeuvres are accompanied by rigorous contraction of abdominal muscles, which puts the bulk of the strain on the stomach muscles rather than on the back.

I begin my exercise program with a few of the easier manoeuvres, gradually working up to the more demanding ones, then tapering off with easier routines. I think it's a good idea to begin and end your session with the deep breathing exercise, and to lie in a comfortable position and relax completely for five minutes or so at the end of the program.

AUXILIARY EXERCISES

In addition to the foregoing, there are several beneficial exercises that can be done at various times of the day from a sitting or standing position. These include knee bends, shoulder shrugs (raising shoulders and circling them slowly forwards and backwards), head circling, and elbow touches (with arms at shoulder height, touching elbows together in front and then bringing them as close together as possible behind your back). I find these auxiliary exercises invaluable, particularly when circumstances force me to sit for prolonged periods.

Last summer, for example, Bill and I motored across Canada, and I often wondered whether people in passing cars were chuckling at that crazy lady in the passenger seat of our van doing shoulder shrugs or head circles! These routines also come in handy at the office. During each four-hour shift at work I try to take time to do a few knee bends, shoulder shrugs, and elbow touches. It's better than a coffee break!

Here, again, I have purposely omitted detailed instructions and diagrams. Rather, I suggest you ask your clinician about some auxiliary exercises that would be suitable for you.

You may feel that some of the exercises described in this brief summary of advanced and auxiliary routines don't apply to you since they aren't specifically aimed at the back and its supporting muscles. But everyone, particularly osteoporotics, should strive to keep *all* their muscles in top shape.

I regularly use the pelvic tilt to relieve back strain when either standing or sitting for prolonged periods. In addition to its therapeutic effect, this exercise has the added advantage of being unobtrusive. While you might feel somewhat reluctant to be seen doing shoulder shrugs or elbow touches at your desk or in a social setting, you can do as many pelvic tilts as you like, and no one will be any the wiser.

WALKING AND SWIMMING

Because walking is often the first exercise an osteoporotic patient can do, and because it is safe for everyone, I think it falls into a special category. Whatever other exercise regimen is prescribed for you, you should try to walk for at least half an hour a day. Of course, if you're still in the acute phase of disability you won't be able to manage this all at once, but you can make it up by several five-minute strolls either indoors or out.

That's the way I started, although at first I was convinced I'd never again make it around a city block. Now I can hike up to five miles if allowed a couple of short rests along the way. And if I can do it, you can too. So persevere. The ultimate reward is well worth the effort.

Swimming, while an excellent overall body toner that doesn't put undue strain on the skeleton, can't be classified as a weight-bearing exercise. So don't substitute swimming for walking. Both have their place in your exercise program, but of the two, I'd say walking is the more important if increasing bone mass is part of your goal.

SUMMARY

It would be difficult to overstate the role exercise has played in my return to near-normal mobility. My muscles are stronger now than they were before the vertebral fractures occurred. I used to be subject to aches and pains in the arms and shoulders attributed to bursitis or some similar cause. I have had no such trouble in the past six years. My legs, too, are much stronger, and I have no difficulty doing deep knee bends, or squatting to perform various gardening and household chores. In short, apart from the weakness and occasional pain attributable to a damaged spine, I feel I'm in great shape (figuratively speaking, of course!).

Whatever your age and condition, there is some form of exercise routine that will be suitable and helpful for you. It's up to you to find it. The first step is to locate a physiotherapist who thoroughly understands your condition and with whom you have a good rapport.

Once you and your therapist have established a suitable program, it should become as much a part of your daily routine as brushing your teeth. I don't let holidays or visitors interfere with my exercise regimen, although I must confess to sometimes doing a slightly pared-down version when travelling. But I do make sure I walk whenever we stop to fill the gas tank or for a lunch or coffee break. And an evening stroll is always part of our travelling routine.

This chapter has been specifically aimed at osteoporotics. Nonetheless, I hope any readers who, happily, don't fall into that category will be encouraged to establish their own exercise program as a vital part of the defensive mechanism. Even if sports are already a major part of your routine, I would recommend at least 15 minutes a day of calisthenics specifically aimed at the back and supporting musculature. Such a regimen could well ward off future problems in this area, whether from osteoporosis or from other causes.

Chapter 7
Support
Organizations

My initial attempts early in 1982 to find information on osteoporosis, this strange affliction that had seemingly struck out of the blue, ran into a virtual blank wall. I didn't know then that organizations were already forming in Ontario that would, in the course of the next couple of years, turn this discouraging situation around.

The summer of 1982 saw the birth of the Osteoporosis Society of Canada. This society, established to serve the needs and interests of those affected by osteoporosis, is a fully registered charitable organization. Its aims, as outlined in an excellent brochure entitled "Osteoporosis: The Silent Thief," are "to focus attention on the problems of this bone condition, to inform both the public and health professionals of the advances in patient treatment and to encourage and support research."

The fact that the first brochure produced by the Osteoporosis Society, "Osteoporosis 'Back to Basics'," had a distribution of some 10,000 copies is evidence of the crying need for such an organization. Since then the Society has been instrumental in instituting a patient rehabilitation program at Toronto's Queen Elizabeth Hospital, in co-sponsoring symposia on osteoporosis, and in preparing video tapes and printed material for use in patient rehabilitation and public awareness programs. Their newsletter, "Osteoporosis Update" and their series "Bulletin for Physicians," keep both the public and doctors informed of new developments.

The Society's medical advisory board consists of some 20 doctors from across the country who collectively represent a formidable array of medical credentials. Free information brochures are available from the Society's national office, or any of the volunteer chapters now being organized across Canada. This service is provided through the donations they are able to raise from individuals and corporations. The address of the Osteoporosis Society of Canada is given at the end of this chapter, along with those of the Canadian self-help groups and various bodies in the United States dealing with osteoporosis.

The stated purpose of the National Osteoporosis Foundation in the United States is very similar to that of the Osteoporosis Society of Canada, namely:

To reduce widespread incidence of osteoporosis through

1. increasing public awareness and knowledge of osteoporosis;
2. providing information to victims;
3. educating physicians and allied healthcare professionals;
4. advocating increased government support for research, and
5. supporting basic research.

Founded in 1986, the Foundation is developing a nationwide support network of regional chapters. A $20 donation per year is requested for individual membership. Anyone interested in organizations in the United States will be able to obtain information by writing to one of the addresses listed at the end of the chapter, or through contact with health-related groups in individual states.

The first Canadian self-help group for osteoporosis, Ostop Ontario (since renamed Ostop Ottawa), took its fledgling steps in the autumn of 1981 under the caring guidance of Lindy Fraser, a dynamic octogenarian from Ottawa who had suffered from osteoporosis for decades. Her continuing battle against the ravages of the disorder is an unusual, perhaps a unique, story which can best be told in her own words. The following is an excerpt from her Christmas 1983 letter.

> . . . I have had osteoporosis for many years, but as I never found a doctor who could diagnose my trouble, I just tried to live with an unknown disease. It had begun when I was young, grew steadily worse, until at the age of 52 I was becoming crippled and deformed, suffering terrible pain, and was forced in 1946 to give up my job as a seed analyst in Winnipeg.

Then in 1947, soon after moving to Gull Lake, I frac-
tured my hip, and went to the nearest doctor 26 miles
away in the little town of Beausejour (Manitoba) where
a young doctor—Dr. Brooks—told me I had osteo-
porosis. I had never heard the name, but it was good
to know that my many years of suffering had a name.
Sadly, Dr. Brooks had to tell me that there was no
treatment available for the disease.

. . . I had to wait many more years before help came.
I became very badly crippled, deformed and hopeless.
Finally, in the late fifties, doctors had learned how to
use calcium for osteoporosis. I responded to the treat-
ment, but it was slow work, as my body was so riddled
with the disease I had little left to fight with. I struggled
along from one fracture to another, in and out of hos-
pital for weeks at a time, until finally, in 1973, my
specialist had to tell me there was nothing more they
could do for me.

. . . By chance, I heard that a doctor in the Ottawa
Civic Hospital, where I was a patient, was part of a
team of researchers testing a new drug for treatment
of osteoporosis. I asked to see this doctor, and
Dr. John Gay very graciously came to tell me about
this trial drug. He thought that sodium fluoride,
combined with calcium, might be a successful treat-
ment for osteoporosis.

Most willingly I began this trial of treatment. We
both knew it would be a long, slow, and very difficult
task. That was in 1973. I was 79 years old. With
wonderful help from many great people, the miracle
happened. It took me a year to get out of bed. I had
to work hard to get into a wheelchair and even harder
to get out of it. I learned to walk again for the third
time, and the wonder of that time has never left me.

I first contacted Lindy Fraser in 1983 after having seen her
on the CBC program "The Nature of Things." Her response was
immediate, the first real encouragement I had had in fighting my
own battle with osteoporosis. Lindy and I became firm long-
distance friends. Whenever I felt disposed to skip my daily walk,
I'd think of this gutsy octogenarian putting in two miles a day

through the corridors of her high-rise apartment when inclement weather kept her indoors. Lindy is more than thirty years my senior. The inspiration of her courageous life has been a constant morale booster.

I was thrilled when, in July 1984, I was well enough to travel to Ottawa and meet my friend face to face. That meeting was like a reunion of kindred spirits. We found we had much in common besides our crooked backs—similar tastes in books and music, for example, and a similar philosophy of life.

When you're in the presence of this four-foot, seven-inch bundle of energy you tend to forget her deformity and the pain she must be suffering. You are conscious only of her vitality, her keen, penetrating glance, the depth of her intelligence, and her total dedication. We spent a delightful day together going over her voluminous material on osteoporosis, chatting about this and that, taking pictures, and comparing wardrobes. I left her with great reluctance, but with renewed courage to persevere with my own project—this book.

Lindy's prime interest was to foster self-help groups for osteoporotics. She gives the following compelling reasons for establishing and/or attending such groups.

1. Sharing experiences.
2. Helper therapy ("Helping you—Helps me" theory).
3. Ideology (belief system). To move out of a state of despair and learn to cope.
4. Network of peers.
5. Sense of equal participation.
6. Source of information re condition or problem.
7. Doctors could find such groups a vital source of information.
8. Advocacy role. Groups can lobby governments whereas individuals would find this difficult.

She began by advertising her plans in Ottawa papers, and things snowballed from there. Medical people contacted her, as did radio and television interviewers, attracted no doubt by her unique history. She was soon addressing interested groups both large and small, and taping material for radio and television. In addition to newspaper coverage, Lindy was featured in three glossy magazine articles in one year.

She and her group were already becoming well known in Ontario when, in the fall of 1982, she appeared with Dr. David Suzuki, noted Canadian geneticist and broadcaster, on the CBC program "The Nature of Things." This appearance sparked a nationwide breakthrough. Says Lindy, "That show brought a phenomenal response in letters of enquiry, which still continue to come." There were thousands of people desperately in need of help. No doubt this nationwide coverage had much to do with the success of Lindy's efforts to get self-help groups organized. There are now active groups in Vancouver, Victoria, and Ottawa.

All these groups provide their members with factual information on osteoporosis, as well as supplying the moral support so vital in dealing with the psychological aspects of the disorder. They bring in speakers from all branches of the medical and related professions—doctors, nurses, nutritionists, therapists, pharmacists, researchers. They co-operate in staging symposia featuring panels of experts in the field. Some conduct exercise sessions with the supervision of trained professionals. They send out interesting newsletters. In short, the self-help groups give their members the support and encouragement they need to fight their individual battles against osteoporosis, and, equally important, they play a major role in promoting public awareness of this devastating affliction.

While researching this book, I had the privilege of meeting the founders of Ostop B.C. and of the then active Regina Osteoporosis Group. These women—Janet Beadnell and Jean Acton in Regina and Gerda Todd in Vancouver—are, like Lindy Fraser, dedicated to their cause.

In 1984 I attended a symposium in Victoria, a co-operative venture of the University of Victoria, Sandoz Canada Inc., and Ostop B.C. I was greatly impressed not only by the quality of the presentations, but by the fact that all sessions were fully booked weeks in advance—ample evidence that word is spreading.

I would strongly urge osteoporosis sufferers and those in the high-risk category, once they have sought qualified medical help, to contact their nearest self-help group. If you aren't close enough to attend meetings, you can at least get on a mailing list. Membership fees are minimal, and most of the groups are registered charitable organizations, so that fees and/or contributions are income tax deductible.

Perhaps you'll even be inspired to organize a self-help group in your own community. Lindy Fraser had much sound advice to offer in this regard. I quote from her circular, "Ideas on Setting Up a Self-help Group":

> *I would want a self-help group to be autonomous of the organizer. In other words it should, from the first, build heavily on the experience of members and their knowledge. As organizer I would work from my own base of experience, always with the insistence that the group must feel they are a GROUP to help each other, and each give of the talents she/he possesses. . . .*
>
> *It is important to set goals and phase each stage slowly and with great care. The first thing is to get together, talk things over, get really acquainted with the idea that each belongs to the other. . . . As organizer I like to keep the feelings of the group in the forefront.*

As a first step, take advantage of any outlets for free advertising that exist in your community. Many radio stations and newspapers provide space for public service announcements, as do some cable television stations. Then there are bulletin boards in supermarkets, laundromats, public buildings, etc. You might ask permission to put material or posters in doctors' offices, medical clinics, and laboratories. News items in local papers can be invaluable.

Most important, get to know others with a similar interest in forming a group, so that you may share the burden of organization. And if you can get the support of some medical people, you'll have won half the battle. Maybe you'll find, as Lindy Fraser did, that you've started a whole new career that will add another dimension to your life. The organizations listed below can provide further tips on getting started.

106

ADDRESSES OF SUPPORT ORGANIZATIONS (CANADA)

Osteoporosis Society of Canada
Ste. 502
76 St. Clair Ave. W.
Toronto, Ont.
M4V 1N2

Osteoporosis Society of Canada
Alberta Chapter
P.O. Box 226
339 – 10 Ave. S.E.
Calgary, Alta.
T2G 0W2

Osteoporosis Society of Canada
Manitoba Chapter
P.O. Box 2099
Winnipeg, Man.
R3C 3R4

Osteoporosis Society of Canada
Quebec Chapter
Penthouse 2
2170 Lincoln Ave.
Montreal, Quebec
H3H 2N5

Ostop Ottawa
c/o Good Companions Centre
670 Albert St.
Ottawa, Ont.
K1R 6L2

Ostop Society of B.C.
203 – 2182 12th Ave. W.
Vancouver, B.C.
V6K 2N4

Ostop Society of B.C.
Victoria Group
841 Fairfield Rd.
Victoria, B.C.
V8V 3B6

ADDRESSES OF SUPPORT ORGANIZATIONS (U.S.A.)

National Osteoporosis Foundation
1625 Eye St. N.W., Ste. 822
Washington, DC 20006
(Steering Committees are working to form new chapters in Georgia, Ohio, Missouri, Colorado, and California.)

National Institute of Arthritis and Musculoskeletal
    and Skin Diseases
National Institutes of Health
Bethesda, MD 20892

Osteoporosis Awareness Resource
c/o Vern Jenkins, R.P.T.
2022 West Weile Ave.
Spokane, WA 99208

Shasta County Awareness Group
c/o Helen Fisher
3304 – 48 Shasta Dam Blvd.
Central Valley, CA 96019

Conclusion

While I have tried to write in an optimistic vein, I do not want to give the impression that osteoporosis is a minor, or even a curable, condition. It is a serious medical problem and one which is likely to affect increasing numbers as the baby boom generation ages. In 1985, the United States Congress declared May 1 through 7 National Osteoporosis Awareness week. The fact that the National Osteoporosis Foundation has made this an annual event (renamed National Osteoporosis Prevention Week in 1987) is ample evidence of the growing concern in North America.

Although there has been considerable progress in various aspects of research in recent years, early diagnosis and screening of at-risk patients remains a problem. There is a continuing lack, particularly in smaller centres, of readily available and affordable methods of accurately measuring bone mass. This makes it difficult to assess the efficacy of any treatment regimen.

On the medical front, there is a continuing need for research to solve these problems, and a corresponding need for greater funding from both government and private sources. There is also a need for general practitioners to take a more active role in advising patients about diet and exercise as preventive measures. It is vital, once the condition has been diagnosed, that much greater attention be paid to exercise, with guidance from a trained therapist continuing until the patient reaches her peak level.

There is also a need for a more informed public, so that women, young and old alike, might look to their defences. But, human nature being what it is, the process of prevention through education and individual action is likely to take a long time.

In the meantime, I hope that this little volume will be of some help to patients already suffering the ravages of osteoporosis. It is to this end that I have written at such length about my personal experience with the condition. I realize that each patient is unique and that all may not achieve the same measure of recovery. However, with a knowledgeable and understanding doctor to prescribe medication, with a competent therapist to direct the all-important exercise program, and, perhaps even more important, with determination and perseverance on the part of the patient, great progress can be made.

My friend Lindy Fraser, who didn't hit upon this happy combination until her 80th year, is living proof that age needn't be a deterrent. Now 94 years old, Lindy is enjoying retirement in a seniors' complex in Ottawa. Unfortunately, she is no longer able to take an active role in Ostop but is content that the organization has reached maturity under the professional guidance of the first executive, which she chose in 1983.

In May of 1985, Lindy was one of the recipients of the "Lifestyle Award," conferred that year by the Honourable Jake Epp, Canada's Health and Welfare Minister at the time. This award is given in recognition of volunteer work in the area of health and social services. Lindy was given special recognition for having performed this service at such an advanced age. She was 91 when the award was conferred. Earlier in the same year, filming began for a half-hour documentary, on the life and times of Lindy Fraser, called "Yes—You Can." The final segment of this film was footage from the award ceremony in May, and was produced by Crawley Films in collaboration with Health and Welfare Canada and the Secretary of State. This film is a tribute to Lindy's fighting spirit. Its focus is an interview in her apartment, but it also shows her shopping and taking the bus to attend Ostop Ottawa meetings. Groups interested in screening the film may contact Hector Balthazar, Canadian Council on Social Development, telephone: (613) 728-1865.

Lindy Fraser's example can give all osteoporosis sufferers, whatever their age or condition, the courage to persevere in their personal battles with the disease. Maybe some happy day researchers will come up with a fool-proof screening and diagnostic method. Maybe they'll find a miracle cure. But in the meantime, it's up to us, the victims or potential victims of the bone robber, to take a hand in our own defence.

Bibliography

Preface and Introduction

Ashpole, Barry R. "Bone Disease Gains Higher Profile in the Minds of Health Care Professionals and the General Public." *Therapeutic Update* (1984): 2,1.

Heaney, Dr. Robert P. "Osteoporosis: An Overview." *Therapeutic Update* (1984): 2,2.

Kaplan, Frederick S., M.D. *Clinical Symposia (Osteoporosis)*. Mississauga, Ontario: CIBA Pharmaceutical Company, 1983.

Osteoporosis Society of Canada. Circular letter, November 1987.

Walker, Dr. V. R. "Osteoporosis, Problems and Treatment of This Bone-losing Disease." *Drug Merchandising* (1983): 64,6.

Ziloski, Mark, M.D. and Morrow, Lewis B., M.D. "Osteoporosis." *Practical Therapeutics* December 1987.

Chapter 2

Ashpole, Barry R. "Bone Disease Gains Higher Profile in the Minds of Health Care Professionals and the General Public." *Therapeutic Update* (1984): 2,1.

American Medical Association Book of Back Care. New York: Random House, 1982.

Harrison, Dr. J. E.; Murray, Dr. T. M.; and Bright-See, Dr. E. eds. "Recent Advances in Osteoporosis." *Clinical and Investigative Medicine* (1982): 5,2/3.

Harsanyi, Dr. Zsolt and Hutton, Richard. *Genetic Prophecy: Beyond the Double Helix*. New York: Rawson Wade, 1982.

Heaney, Dr. Robert P. "Osteoporosis: An Overview." *Therapeutic Update* (1984): 2,2.

Inglis, Brian. *The Book of the Back*. New York: Hearst Books, 1978.

Kaplan, Frederick S., M.D. *Clinical Symposia (Osteoporosis)*. Mississauga, Ontario: CIBA Pharmaceutical Company, 1983.

Mayes, Kathleen. *Osteoporosis: Brittle Bones and the Calcium Crisis.* Santa Barbara: Pennant Books, 1986.

Melleby, Alexander. *The Y's Way to a Healthy Back.* Piscataway, N.J.: New Century, 1982.

Michele, Arthur A., M.D. *Orthotherapy.* New York: M. Evans, 1971.

"Osteoporosis: Fear of Falling." *Health News* (1984): 2,1.

Raisz, Lawrence G., M.D. "Osteoporosis." Presented at the White House Conference on Aging, November 1981.

Riggs, B. Lawrence, M.D. and Melton, L. Joseph III, M.D. "Evidence for Two Distinct Syndromes of Involutional Osteoporosis." *The American Journal of Medicine* (1983): 75.

Root, Leon, M.D. and Kiernan, Thomas. *Oh, My Aching Back.* New York: David McKay, 1973.

Smith, Everett L., Ph.D. "Exercise for Prevention of Osteoporosis: A Review." *The Physician and Sports Medicine* (1982): 10,3.

Smith, Wendy. *Osteoporosis—How to Prevent the Brittle Bone Disease.* New York: Simon and Schuster, 1985.

Walker, Dr. V. R. "Osteoporosis, Problems and Treatment of This Bone-losing Disease." *Drug Merchandising* (1983): 64,6.

Chapter 3

Anderson, C.; Cape, R.D.T.; Crilly, R. G.; Hodsman, A. B.; and Wolfe, B. M. "Preliminary Observations of a Form of Coherence Therapy for Osteoporosis." *Calcified Tissue International* (Springer-Verlag) (1984).

Ashpole, Barry R. "Bone Disease Gains Higher Profile in the Minds of Health Care Professionals and the General Public." *Therapeutic Update* (1984): 2,1.

Banna, M., Associate Professor of Neuroradiology, McMaster University, Hamilton, Ont. "The CT Scan." Undated paper.

Bayley, T. A.; Harrison, J. E.; Josse, R. G.; Murray, T. M.; Sturtridge, W.; Williams, C.; Patt, N.; Goodwin, S.; Pritzker, K.; and Fornasier, V. (Bone and Mineral Group, University of Toronto, St. Joseph's Health Centre, Toronto General, St. Michael's, Mt. Sinai, Wellesley and Queen Elizabeth Hospitals, Toronto.) "The Relationships Between Fluoride Effects on Bone Histology, Bone Mass, and

Bone Strength." Paper presented at the International Symposium on Osteoporosis, Denmark, 1987.

"Biomedical Imaging Director Invents Device to Detect Osteoporosis." *Insider Bulletin* 8 April 1988.

Budden, F. H.; Bayley, T. A.; Harrison, J. E.; Josse, R. G.; Murray, T. M.; Sturtridge, W. C.; Kandel, R.; Vieth, R.; Strauss, A. L.; and Goodwin, S. "The Effect of Fluoride on Bone Histology in Post-menopausal Osteoporosis Depends on Adequate Fluoride Absorption and Retention." *Journal of Bone and Mineral Research* (1988): 3,2.

"Building Up Brittle Bones." *Time* 7 December 1981.

Chow, Dr. Raphael; Harrison, Dr. Joan; Dornan, Dr. James. "The P.R.O. (Prevention and Rehabilitation of Osteoporosis) Program." Paper presented at the 6th International Symposium on Adapted Physical Activity, Brisbane, Australia, June 1987.

Chow, Raphael; Harrison, Joan E.; Notarius, Cathy. "Effect of Two Randomised Exercise Programmes on Bone Mass of Healthy Post-Menopausal Women." *British Medical Journal* 5 December 1987.

Christiansen, C.; Riis, B. J.; and Rødbro, P. "Prediction of Rapid Bone Loss in Postmenopausal Women." *The Lancet* 16 May 1987.

Dixon, Allan St. J. "Non-hormonal Treatment of Osteoporosis." *British Medical Journal* (1983): 286,6370.

Doppelt, Dr. Samuel. "Osteoporosis—A Silent Epidemic." *The Medical Forum* (November 1981).

Evasuk, Stasia. "Bone Disease Experiment Needs Women for Class." *Toronto Star* 7 June 1984.

Goltzman, David. "Osteoporosis." *Medicine North America* 15 September 1984.

Grove, O. and Halver, B. "Relief of Osteoporotic Backache with Fluoride, Calcium, and Calciferol." *Acta Medica Scandinavica*: 209,6.

Hangartner, T. N.; Overton, T. R.; Harley, C. H.; Berg, L. van den; and Crockford, P. M. "Skeletal Challenge: An Experimental Study of Pharmacologically Induced Changes in Bone Density in the Distal Radius, Using Gamma-ray Computed Tomography." *Calcified Tissue International* (1985).

Hangartner, Thomas N. and Overton, Thomas R. "Quantitative Measurement of Bone Density Using Gamma-ray Computed Tomography." *Journal of Computer Assisted Tomography* (1982) 6(6): 1156-1162.

Harrison, J. E.; Bayley, T. A.; Josse, R. G.; Murray, T. M.; Sturtridge, W.; Williams, C.; Goodwin, S.; Tam, C.; and Fornasier, V. "The Relationship Between Fluoride Effects on Bone Histology and on Bone Mass in Patients with Postmenopausal Osteoporosis." *Bone and Mineral*, 1 (1986): 321-33.

Harrison, J. E.; McNeill, K. G.; Sturtridge, W. C.; Bayley, T. A.; Murray, T. M.; Williams, C.; Tam, C.; and Fornasier, V. "Three-year Changes in Bone Mineral Mass of Postmenopausal Osteoporotic Patients Based on Neutron Activation Analysis of the Central Third of the Skeleton." *Journal of Clinical Endocrinology and Metabolism* (1981): 52,4.

Harrison, Dr. J. E.; Murray, Dr. T. M.; and Bright-See, Dr. E. eds. "Recent Advances in Osteoporosis." *Clinical and Investigative Medicine* (1982): 5,2,3.

Heaney, Dr. Robert P. "Osteoporosis: An Overview." *Therapeutic Update* (1984): 2,2.

Jenkins, Kristin. "Osteoporosis Rivals Dementia as Most Serious Problem of Old Age." *Ontario Medicine* 15 August 1983.

Josse, Robert G., M.B., F.R.C.P.(C), F.A.C.P. "Drug Treatment of Osteoporosis." *Drug Protocol* (1988): 3,5.

Josse, Robert G. "Osteoporosis: An Update on Pathogenesis and Treatment." *Canadian Family Physician* (1983): 29.

Kaplan, Frederick S., M.D. *Clinical Symposia (Osteoporosis)*. Mississauga, Ontario: CIBA Pharmaceutical Company, 1983.

Mayes, Kathleen. *Osteoporosis: Brittle Bones and the Calcium Crisis*. Santa Barbara: Pennant Books, 1986.

Notelovitz, Morris, M.D. and Ware, Marsha. *Stand Tall! Every Woman's Guide to Preventing Osteoporosis*. Gainesville, Florida: Triad, 1982; New York: Bantam Books, 1985.

"Osteoporosis: Fear of Falling." *Health News* (1984): 2,1.

"Osteoporosis Is Not a Normal Ageing Process." *Therapeutic Update* January 1983.

Payer, Lynn. "Daily Calcium Levels May Have Been Set Too Low."
Medical Post 30 June 1981.

Raisz, Lawrence, M.D. "Osteoporosis." Presented at the White House
Conference on Aging, November 1981.

Recker, Robert R. "Osteoporosis." *Contemporary Nutrition* (1983): 5.

Reginster, J.Y. et al. "One-year Controlled Randomized Trial of Prevention of Early Post-Menopausal Bone Loss by Inter-nasal Calcitonin." *The Lancet* 26 December 1987.

"Results with Sodium Fluoride in Osteoporosis Encouraging." *Ontario
Medicine* 9 July 1984.

Riggs, B. Lawrence, M.D.; Seeman, Ego, M.D.; Hodgson, Stephen
F., M.D.; Taves, Donald R., M.D.; and O'Fallon, W. Michael,
Ph.D. "Effect of the Fluoride/Calcium Regimen on Vertebral Frac-
ture Occurrence in Postmenopausal Osteoporosis." *The New
England Journal of Medicine* 25 February 1982.

Riggs, B. Lawrence, M.D. and Melton, Joseph III, M.D. "Evidence
for Two Distinct Syndromes of Involutional Osteoporosis." *The
American Journal of Medicine* (1983): 75.

Silburt, Dave. "Osteoporosis Research Aimed at Prevention." *RPC*
September 1984.

Sutton, Dr. Roger and Gibson, Dr. Morris. Interview. "Best Catch
Osteoporosis Before First Fracture." *The Medical Post* 2 October
1984.

Ziloski, Mark, M.D. and Morrow, Lewis B., M.D. "Osteoporosis."
Practical Therapeutics December 1987.

Chapter 4

Hall, Hamilton, M.D. *The Back Doctor*. Toronto: MacMillan of
Canada, 1980.

Chapter 5

Albanese, Anthony A., Ph.D. "Calcium Nutrition in the Elderly."
Postgraduate Medicine (1978): 63,3.

Bright-See, Dr. Elizabeth. "Bone Up on Your Calcium Needs." *Canadian Living* (1984): 9,9.

Brody, Jane. "Milk: Make No Bones about It." *The Province*
17 January 1984.

Calcium: A Summary of Current Research for the Health Professional. Rosemount, Illinois: National Dairy Council, 1984.

"Calcium Supplements with a Touch of Lead." *Consumer Reports* September 1982.

Coleman, Lester L., M.D. "Yogurt Can Help Lactose Intolerance." *Vernon Daily News* 16 August 1984.

"Diet and Osteoporosis." In *Osteoporosis, How to Cope.* Osteoporosis Society of Canada.

Forster-Coull, E. "Diet and Osteoporosis." A Review Paper, April 1984.

Fujita, Takuo, M.D. *Calcium and Your Health.* Briarcliff Manor, N.Y.: Japan Publications, 1987.

Hay, J. K. "Calcium Compounds for Treating Osteoporosis." *Canadian Family Physician* February 1984.

Hope, Jane and Bright-See, Dr. Elizabeth. "Steps to Help You Ward Off Osteoporosis." *The Toronto Star* 21 November 1984.

"Important Points to Remember in Counseling Patients Who Use Oral Calcium Supplements." *Canadian Pharmaceutical Journal* April (1987).

Isogna, Dr. Karl L. "Antacid Can Cause Bone Pain and Deterioration." *Journal of the American Medical Association* 5 December 1980.

Like Mother, Like Daughter: A Mature Woman's Guide to Bone Health. Rosemount, Illinois: National Dairy Council, 1984.

Mann, Peggy. "Teenagers and the Calcium Crisis." *The Saturday Evening Post* April 1987.

Matkovic, V., M.D., Ph.D. In "Teenagers and the Calcium Crisis." *The Saturday Evening Post* April 1987.

McCarron, D. A.; Chesnut, C. H.; Cob, C.; and Baylink, D. J. "Blood Pressure Response to Pharmacologic Management of Osteoporosis." *Clinical Research* (1981): 29,274A.

McCarron, D. A.; Morris, C. D.; and Cole, C. "Dietary Calcium in Human Hypertension." *Science* (1982): 217,267-269.

Mowbray, Scott. "The Educated Eater." *Western Living* October 1984.

Murray, Timothy, M.D. "Osteoporosis—The Importance of Nutrition for Healthy Bones." *Nutrition Quarterly* (1983): 7,4.

Nakai, Shuryo. "Can Cow's Milk Prevent Disease?" *Nutrition Quarterly* (1983): 7,4.

Notelovitz, M., M.D. and Ware, Marsha. *Stand Tall! Every Woman's Guide to Preventing Osteoporosis.* Gainesville, Florida: Triad, 1982; New York, Bantam Books, 1985.

"Nutrient Value of Some Common Foods." Health and Welfare Canada 1979.

"Osteoporosis." *Consumer Reports* (1984): 49,10.

"Osteoporosis: Fear of Falling." *Health News* (1984): 2,1.

"Osteoporosis Is Not a Normal Ageing Process." *Therapeutic Update.* January 1983.

Payer, Lynn. "Daily Calcium Levels May Have Been Set Too Low." *Medical Post* 30 June 1981.

Recker, Robert R., M.D. "The Role of Calcium in Bone Health." *Nutrition News* (1984): 47,2.

Recker, Robert R., M.D. "Osteoporosis." *Contemporary Nutrition* (1983): 5.

"The Role of Calcium in Health." *Dairy Council Digest* (1984): 55,1.

Seeman, E., M.D. and Riggs, B. L., M.D. "Dietary Factors and Osteoporosis in the Elderly." *Geriatrics* (1981): 36,9.

"Shopping for Food and Nutrition." (Pub. No. 1651) Ottawa: Health and Welfare Canada, 1980.

"Sodium Information Sheet." Rosemount, Illinois: National Dairy Council, 1984.

Spencer, Herta, M.D. and Kramer, Lois, R.D. "Bone Loss with Aging." *Nutrition Quarterly* (1983): 7,4.

Spencer, Herta, M.D.; Kramer, Lois, B.S.; and Osis, Dace. "Factors Contributing to Calcium Loss in Aging." *The American Journal of Clinical Nutrition* (1982): 36.

Spencer, Herta, M.D.; Kramer, Lois, B.S.; DeBartolo, Michele, B.S.; Norris, Clemontain, R.N.; and Osis, Dace. "Further Studies on the Effect of a High Protein Diet as Meat on Calcium Metabolism." *The American Journal of Clinical Nutrition* (1983): 37.

Spencer, Herta, M.D.; Kramer, Lois, B.S.; Norris, Clemontain, R.N.; and Osis, Dace. "Effect of Small Doses of Aluminum-Containing Antacids on Calcium and Phosphorus Metabolism." *The American Journal of Clinical Nutrition* (1982): 36.

"Your Calcium Needs Will Increase with Your Age." Dorval, Quebec: Sandoz (Canada) Inc. Pamphlet, 1984.

Chapter 6

"Back Talk, an Owner's Manual for Backs." Workers' Compensation Board of British Columbia Pamphlet, October 1979.

"*Don't Take it Easy (Fitness for the Older Canadian).*" Ottawa: Dept. of Fitness and Amateur Sport, 1981.

"Osteoporosis." *Consumer Reports* (1984): 49,10.

"Osteoporosis, How to Cope." Osteoporosis Society of Canada Pamphlet.

"Other Factors Affecting Calcium Utilization." In *Calcium: A Summary of Current Research for the Health Professional.* Rosemount, Illinois: National Dairy Council, 1984.

Recker, Dr. Robert R. "Osteoporosis." General Mills Nutrition Dept. (1983): 8,5.

Root, Leon, M.D. and Kiernan, Thomas. *Oh, My Aching Back.* New York: David McKay, 1973.

Smith, Everett L., Ph.D. "Exercise for Prevention of Osteoporosis: A Review." *The Physician and Sports Medicine* (1982): 10,3.

Chapter 7

Fraser, Lindy. "Ideas on Setting Up a Self-help Group." Circular letter, February 1983.

Gregory, Joy. "This Little Old Lady Just Won't Quit." Reader's Digest Assn. (Canada) Ltd., 1986.

Ireland, Cheryllynn. "Lindy Fraser: An Inspiration." *Meridian* October 1986.

"Lindy Fraser Uses Self-help for Osteoporosis Sufferers." *Ottawa Revue* 25 April-1 May 1984.

Lofaro, Tony. "Senior's Long Fight with Bone Disease Subject of Film." *Ottawa Citizen* 17 June 1986.

"The Nature of Things." Transcript of television broadcast. The Canadian Broadcasting Corp. 17 November 1982.

"Osteoporosis, Back to the Basics." Introductory brochure. Osteoporosis Society of Canada. 1982.

"Osteoporosis Society of Canada." Personal letter to author, 9 November 1983.

"Ostop Ontario." Circular letter, December 1983.

"Ostop Ottawa Newsletter." (1983-84): 1,1.

The Ostop Society of B.C. Newsletter. (1984): 1.

"Senior's Group Battles Bone Disease." *The Centretown News* (Ottawa) 21 October 1983.

Index

Note: Tables are not indexed. Doctors mentioned or cited in text are, for your convenience, grouped here under the general heading Doctors.

treatment, 6ff.
urine level, 43-44, 70, 89
Calcium-phosphate ratio, 92
Canes (walking canes, stick chairs),
58
Ca-ph ratio. *See* Calcium-phosphate
ratio
Car seats, 60-61
Causes (of osteoporosis). *See*
Osteoporosis
Cervical vertebrae. *See* Spine
Chairs
footstool, 60
lawn, 59
Obus Forme, 60
rocking, 6-7, 59
secretary's, 59
See also Canes
Cheeses, 74
Chelated calcium supplements.
See Calcium
Chronic glucocorticoid excess.
See Hyperadrenalism
Citrocarbonate. *See* Antacids
Clothing. *See* Personal appearance
Coccyx. *See* Spine
Cocoa mix. *See* Recipes
Coffee. *See* Caffeine
Coherence therapy, 47
Collagen. *See* Dietary factors
(protein)
Compression of organs. *See*
Abdomen
C.T. scan (Quantitative computed
tomography), 41
Cortical bone. *See* Bone
Cortisone, 25
Coughing, 61
Curvature of the spine, 1, 9, 17, 28

Definition of osteoporosis.
See Osteoporosis
Delcid. *See* Antacids
Diabetes, 24
Diagnosis of osteoporosis. *See*
Osteoporosis

Didronel. *See* Sodium
diphosphonate
Dietary factors, 21-22, 26-27
cod-liver oil, 14, 23, 88
dietary analysis, 81-82
milk equivalents to calcium
content, 74
protein, 22, 88
recipes (cocoa mix, yogurt), 75-76
snacks, 75
sodium (salt), 88-91
vitamin A, 88
vitamin C, 88
vitamin D, 6, 23, 36, 87-88
See also Alcohol, Aluminum
compounds, Caffeine,
Calcium, Cheeses, Fibre, Milk,
Oxalates, Phosphates, Tobacco
Di-Gel. *See* Antacids
Disease-induced bone loss.
See Bone
Distal radius (wrist), 4, 27, 41
Doctors
Anderson, C., 47
Anderson, John, 69
Banna, M., 41
Cape, R.D.T., 47
Chow, Raphael, 51-52
Christiansen, Claus, 44
Crilly, R. G., 47
Delmas, P. D., 23
Dornan, James, 51
Fujita, Takuo, 69-70
Gallagher, Chris, 50
Gay, John, 103
Hall, Hamilton, 61
Hangartner, T. N., 41-42
Harrison, Joan, 19-20, 21, 23,
27, 42, 45, 51
Harsanyi, Zsolt, 24
Heaney, Robert P., 21, 22, 47-48
Hodsman, A. B., 47
Hutton, Richard, 24
Insogna, Karl, 25
Josse, Robert G., 50, 52
Kaplan, Frederick S., 18, 19, 20,
22, 23, 25

Urine tests, 6, 43

Vertebrae (anatomy), 28-30
Vitamin A. *See* Dietary factors
Vitamin C. *See* Dietary factors
Vitamin D. *See* Dietary factors

Walking. *See* Exercise
Walking canes or stick chairs.
  See Canes
Wrist. *See* Distal radius

X-rays, 5, 32, 38. *See also*
  Radiogrammetry, Radiographic
  photodensitometry

Yogurt. *See* Recipes